Orthopaedic Appliances

by

BRIAN H. DAY, F.R.C.S.

Consultant Orthopaedic Surgeon
St. Helier Group of Hospitals

With illustrations by Audrey Besterman

Faber & Faber
3 Queen Square
London

First published 1972 by
Faber and Faber Limited
3 Queen Square, London, WC1
ISBN 0 571 09947 5

Printed in Great Britain by
Western Printing Services Ltd, Bristol

Contents

List of Figures

LIST OF FIGURES

7

Preface

The purpose of this book is to describe the appliances readily available and their clinical application. This information, which is not available in book form other than in manufacturers' catalogues, is not taught as an organized subject and many doctors at Houseman and Registrar level may not be aware of the types of appliances made, nor of their clinical use. The book is, therefore, laid out assuming that the diagnosis has been made, but a brief description of each condition is given to bring out the main points of importance when considering a suitable appliance. Appliances are then listed and each criticized in turn. Line drawings have been chosen in preference to photographs, because the essential features can be shown more clearly. It is hoped that in this way the doctor concerned will be able to choose the method of treatment best suited for the particular patient under consideration.

ONE

Cervical Collars

It must be appreciated that absolute immobility of the cervical spine is impossible to achieve with an appliance if pressure necrosis is to be avoided over the many bony prominences at the cephalic end of the collar. Pressure must be taken against the occiput and the lower margin of the mandible, and movement of the latter during eating and talking precludes full support being provided. Similarly, the skin over the clavicles is also at risk at the caudal end of the applicance.

Nevertheless, sufficient support and immobilization can be achieved if one remembers that most cervical collars are prescribed for a lesion which is sited between the 3rd and 7th cervical vertebrae, and it is fortunate that these are the commonest levels at which lesions occur.

Movement of the upper cervical region cannot be prevented unless purchase is taken direct onto the skull and the dorsal vertebrae, and this is obviously not a practical proposition.

When estimating the size of the collar to be worn one must take into account not only the circumference of the neck, but also the distance between the angles of the jaw and the clavicles. Several patterns of cervical collar are in current use, but basically they consist of a relatively rigid, but padded frame encircling the neck and take purchase on the bony points mentioned above.

TEMPORARY COLLAR

A double thickness of sponge rubber or felt wrapped round the neck and bandaged firmly in position provides a reasonable amount of support and certainly restricts movement of the lower cervical spine sufficiently to be of some value until a definitive appliance can be provided. If sheets of adhesive rubber or felt are used it is convenient to fold the sheets, which are supplied by manufacturers in 16 inches × 8 inches (40 × 20 cm.), lengthways, and then to trim the margin as shown in Fig. 1. The material is then enclosed within a length of Tube-gauz which facilitates tying.

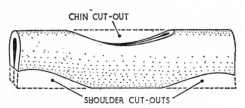

Fig. 1. Temporary cervical collar

INFLATABLE RUBBER COLLAR

This appliance (Fig. 2) consists of three compartments which can be inflated by a common air inlet to any desired tension. The compartments are joined side by side by a strip of rubber, and a flange at either extremity carries laces for adjustment of circumference. By its nature one cannot expect elimination of neck movement but a good deal of support is provided without

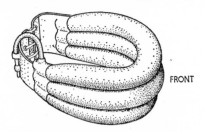

Fig. 2. Inflatable rubber collar

firm edges to cause skin trauma. A considerable disadvantage is the lack of ventilation through the collar and most patients find it uncomfortably hot.

SPONGE RUBBER COLLAR

A sheet of sponge rubber specially shaped to avoid pressure under the clavicles and the end of the chin is enclosed within an envelope of soft leather (Fig. 3). This provides firmer support than an inflatable collar but again suffers from lack of ventilation.

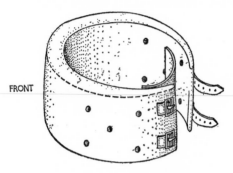

FRONT

Fig. 3. Sponge rubber collar

THOMAS COLLAR

Usually made of a thermo-plastic material and padded with sponge rubber at the upper and lower margins to avoid undue pressure on the jaw and clavicles. As the combination is inherently more rigid than either of those mentioned above,

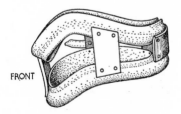

FRONT

Fig. 4. Thomas collar

11

ventilation holes can be cut in the body of the material and for this reason the appliance seems to be more popular with patients than any of those mentioned previously (*see* Fig. 4).

VICTORIA COLLAR

Two strips of spring steel form seven-eighths of a circle; these are suitably padded and connected together by three distance pieces, one in the centre of the curve and one at each extremity (*see* Fig. 5). If these distance pieces are adjusted for height a single collar can be made to fit most people, and therefore one

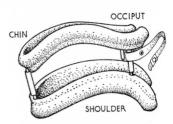

Fig. 5. Victoria collar

stock size usually suffices. One great advantage here is that there is no enclosing material round the neck and patients usually feel more free when using an appliance of this type. Fitting is more comfortable if the upper and lower strips can be bent to encourage pressure to be taken over as large a surface area as possible, but this is not a practical proposition if the upper and lower margins are made of high quality material and therefore resistant to cold bending.

SUMMARY

The above collars all rely on some degree of distraction occurring between the lower margin of the jaw and the clavicles, and although careful shaping can eliminate localized pressure and roughening of the skin, redness over the clavicles and over the angles of the jaw is commonly seen.

FRAME COLLAR

This appliance differs in design from those types mentioned above but the danger of localized pressure on the skin is even greater. The appliance consists of a frame fitting across the shoulders which is made of two strips of steel riveted together at either end, the apices being in the mid-line anteriorly and posteriorly. Each apex is reinforced by a triangular insert of mild steel, that on the dorsal aspect bearing a spring clip. Arising from the dorsal apex is a vertical rod curved to follow the shape of the upper dorsal and the cervical spine. It is hinged

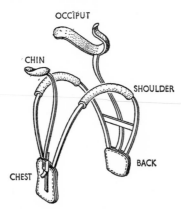

Fig. 6. Frame collar

at its caudal end to the apex of the shoulder frame and bears on its cephalic end a curved strip suitably padded, which bears on the occiput. Its caudal third engages with the spring clip on the triangular insert. Riveted to the anterior apex is a vertical rod bearing at its cephalic end a cupped plate on which the chin rests. In the middle third of this anterior rod it is customary to have a hinge which clips shut to enable the chin support to be dropped forward during application of the collar (*see* Fig. 6).

The fitting of this appliance is very critical if it is to be effective, and one must provide either very careful shaping of the shoulder frame or very thick padding to prevent skin necrosis over the clavicles where these are prominent. Similarly, there is a danger of pressure necrosis over the occiput or point of the chin.

Although this collar does provide considerably more support and control of movement than other types, it can only be worn with loose garments and is much less readily hidden by scarves etc., than those mentioned previously.

DOLL'S COLLAR

This consists of two sheets of thermoplastic material made to a plaster cast of the upper thorax, neck and lower part of the head. Thus a light plaster must be applied first, split down either side, removed from the patient, reassembled and used as a

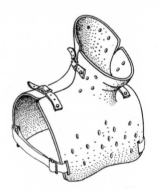

Fig. 7. Doll's collar

negative for a plaster positive, and the thermoplastic material must be moulded to this. It is then split down each lateral margin and suitably padded, the two halves being connected by leather strips and press studs. Reinforcement may be provided and if needed at all it is usually placed down the mid-line anteriorly and posteriorly. In addition to the leather strips and press studs on either side of the head, neck and shoulders a further strap passing through the axilla is provided on either side (*see* Fig. 7).

This appliance provides more control of movement and more support than any of the devices mentioned above, and is by far the most difficult to manufacture and the least comfortable to wear.

TWO

Corsets and Braces

SPINAL APPLIANCES

INTRODUCTION

It is this group of orthopaedic appliances in which one finds the greatest number of inaccurate prescriptions. The reason for this is the failure to understand the indications for the various types of corsets and braces available.

In this book, the corset will be considered as an appliance made of fabric, perhaps with metal stiffeners but without any metal frame which encircles or almost encircles the body. A brace, on the other hand, will be considered as an appliance consisting of a metal frame which encircles or largely encircles the body. This frame may be supplemented by fabric panels, buckles or pads, but the essential feature is that it encircles the body, gaining a firm basis round the pelvis.

FUNCTION

By its nature a corset is unable to provide much corrective force in any direction but relies for its efficiency on the tightness with which it is laced. It is obvious, therefore, that this type of appliance will be inapplicable in many conditions (e.g. pregnancy, hiatus hernia, defects in the diaphragm or in the pelvic floor).

It will also be obvious that because of the lack of a firm basis round the pelvis, a corset will not control body movements as efficiently as will a brace. The appliance will give the patient a feeling of support, a feeling of pressure and will produce a redistribution of body weight.

The redistribution of body weight occurs because of compression of the intra-abdominal contents. The soft abdominal wall is approximated to the more rigid vertebral column, thus displacing the centre of gravity towards the spine. In addition, the compression effect is transmitted to the under surface of the diaphragm and to the upper surface of the pelvic floor and the abdominal cavity is, therefore, lengthened. This effect in itself tends to decrease the ability to flex the spine but the presence of a weak diaphragm or pelvic floor may precipitate herniation through these structures. A tightly laced corset is, therefore, contra-indicated in hiatus hernia, prolapse of the uterus and similar conditions.

CORSETS

Basically, a corset consists of a fabric belt reaching from the level of the symphysis pubis to the costal margin, although this can be extended in a cephalic direction if necessary. It is usual for the front and sides to be stiffened by whalebone or mild steel inserts at intervals of approximately 4 inches (10 cm.) and some form of more rigid metal stiffening is usually present

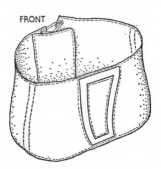

Fig. 8. Goldthwait corset

in the region of the sacro-iliac joints and lumbar spine. In the Goldthwait type of corset, the posterior stiffening consists of a rectangular frame of light metal, some 5 inches (13 cm.) wide at its upper margin and 3 inches (8 cm.) wide over the sacrum, the length of the side bars depending on the height of the corset (*see* Fig. 8).

Other types of appliance, for example the Spencer corset shown in Fig. 9, rely on two longitudinal strips of metal approximately 1 inch (2·5 cm.) wide, which are placed on either side of the mid-line posteriorly. The latter type is less

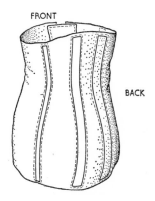

Fig. 9. Spencer corset

restricting in rotation than is the Goldthwait frame but in other aspects there is little to choose between the two.

Forward or lateral flexion is only restricted in these corsets by the tension of the material at the upper margin. It is obvious that if one considers the three-point pressure technique described so well by Charnley in his book *The Closed Treatment of Common Fractures*, one will see that the soft stiffening present in these corsets is insufficient to prevent movement in these directions and it is present simply to prevent the material from rolling up. Flexion of the lumbar spine, therefore, can be limited by extending the corset in a cephalic direction.

Many patients will return, having been supplied with such an appliance, requesting that the upper margin should be cut down since they find there is increased pressure over the costal margin. If this alteration is made, flexion of the lumbar spine is certainly made easier but it is just this movement which one is trying to prevent and it is often wiser to extend the corset 1 inch (2·5 cm.) or 2 inches (5 cm.) higher. This will not only relieve the localized pressure at the costal margin but will render the appliance even more efficient.

It is common, too, to have female patients complaining that a roll of fat is pinched between the upper margin of the corset and the lower margin of the brassière. This effect can be prevented by persuading the patient to wear a brassière which has a deep band below the breasts and this band can be attached to the upper margin of the corset by hooks and eyes or by press-studs.

In either type of corset it is usual to find elastic darts at the sides, and in the Spencer variety, elastic inserts across the fronts of the thighs. These modifications make hip movement easier and patients find that sitting is much more comfortable. Similarly, darts are often inserted laterally at the level of the costal margin since restriction of breathing is less noticed when some elasticity is present.

The opening in a corset may be in the mid-line or one side. The former is usually preferred since most patients tend to assume a central fixing and if this is not supplied, one often finds that the back steels are not symmetrical about the spine.

The method of fastening is unimportant. Lacing is frequently used; this is an extremely efficient method providing very even distribution of the pull but if it is used the laces must be inserted in such a way that they can be tightened at two sites and these sites should be placed on either side of the middle half of the lacing (i.e. one-quarter of the distance down from the top margin and one-quarter of the distance up from the bottom margin). If there is a great deal of lacing left free, this is usually tied into a large bow and pushed back under the free edge of the corset. If this is not done, the bulky knot can be seen through the patient's clothes.

Straps and buckles are also frequently used. If the former are made of fabric, they lie flat against the appliance and are difficult to see through the clothes but if the buckles have prongs, the fabric is damaged and torn by these and frequent replacements of the straps are necessary. Several types of friction buckles are available, the simplest one of which can be tightened simply by pulling the free end of the buckle back towards its fixation point. For loosening this type, the free edge is taken across to the buckle side of the corset, the buckle itself being turned over in the process, and it will then be found that the strap can be slipped back. These buckles lie flat against the skin, are very thin and are only seen under tight dresses.

In addition to the fixation of the main body of the corset, it is common to find a lumbar pad applied either to the outer aspect of the corset or on its inner aspect, the straps arising from it passing through slits in the fabric on either side. In the former case, tightening of these straps ensures that the back steels over the lumbar sacral region are firmly applied to the body, whereas if the lumbar pad is on the inner aspect of the corset, they actually encourage the lumbar steels to lift away from the patient. Thus, if additional local pressure is thought desirable, it should be applied by a supplementary external panel.

When fitting appliances of this nature, it is essential to see that the patient can sit without undue discomfort and that flexion of the spine is limited. One should note the upper margins of all stiffeners and ensure that they do not coincide with any bony prominence. The most common site for pressure is the stiffening on either side of the front lacing or the inserts lateral to these. The upper margin frequently impinges on the costal cartilages and it is common to see a small brown stain on the skin of those patients who have worn corsets of this nature for any length of time; this is most noticeable in females. The solution is to provide the patient with a corset one or two inches higher and to persuade her to wear a brassière with a deep band, which should be put on before the corset is donned.

It is essential to see that the posterior steels are shaped to the curve of the body. One often finds fitters attempting to make the patient fit the corset, rather than the reverse. In Spencer type corsets, it is usually possible to remove the posterior steels and to shape them to the patient before reinserting them in the garment. This ensures a close fit but it is often difficult to assess the position the steel will occupy when the corset is being worn.

Some manufacturers line the back of the corset with padded material under the posterior steels; this is probably a little more comfortable for the patient but it does make accurate curving of the posterior steels more difficult, although one can achieve an extremely good fit with practice.

CONCLUSIONS

It will be seen, therefore, that when providing appliances for low lumbar, lumbo-sacral or sacro-iliac disorders, the main aims are to restrict movement rather than prevent it, and to provide some feeling of support. An appliance of the types described above could be, if carefully fitted, very satisfactory. Indeed, it is much more common to provide appliances of this nature than to order one of the more elaborate braces to be described later.

SPINAL BRACES

For the purpose of this book, a brace is considered as a spinal appliance consisting of a metal frame which wholly or largely encircles the pelvis with metal extensions in various directions according to the particular function of that appliance. The important feature, however, is the fact that the brace almost encircles the body at the level of the pelvis and it is because of firm strapping at this site that a good grip on the body can be achieved and supportive or corrective forces applied elsewhere.

One must accept that complete support or complete limitation of movement of the spine is impossible from a practical point of view for the following reasons:

Direct fixation to bone is impossible and movement of the soft tissues between the appliance and skeleton cannot be prevented. This movement can be decreased considerably if the pressure of the appliance can be concentrated on small areas but if this is done, the skin is unable to withstand the forces applied to it and becomes abraded or, in extreme cases, undergoes pressure necrosis. For practical purposes, therefore, one has to accept a compromise between relative efficiency and the ability of the skin to withstand the pressures applied to it.

Many attempts have been made to design a corrective brace which relies on tension produced in the spine by head traction. If the patient is to be mobile while wearing such an appliance, counter-pressure must be applied to the pelvis and the skin over the iliac crests cannot bear the strains imposed.

In any case, correction of a curve of any mobile structure cannot be done efficiently by increasing the tension applied to that structure. (Note, for example, the curve of telephone wires or of high tension cables between pylons.)

On the other hand, correction of a curve in a structure can be achieved by three-point pressure as is well described in Charnley's book.

For these reasons, therefore, attempts at providing correction by tension have been abandoned and one relies now on direct pressure.

Two basic types of spinal braces are available. They are those that support and those that correct.

MECHANICS OF SPINAL SUPPORTING BRACE

A firm foundation must be achieved and in all types of brace, use is made of firm strapping round the pelvis, just above the greater trochanters. This usually consists of a metal strap hinged to a lumbar frame and there is frequently a second strap hinged to this frame posteriorly, which arches forward above the iliac crest and then curves down to join the first strap in the region of the anterior superior iliac spines. From this basis, a frame usually extends up the spine as far as required and this is known as the back lever. Extending from this are bars or straps which encircle the shoulders and this combination can be seen greatly to restrict the flexion of the lumbar spine.

It is common to add a fabric support encircling the abdomen. This has the same effect as a corset, as described above, in that it shifts the centre of gravity towards the spine and also gives some support by the effect of transmission of the pressure of abdominal contents to the under-surface of the diaphragm.

INDIVIDUAL APPLIANCES

MCKEE BRACE

This consists of a rectangular posterior frame extending from the first or second part of the sacrum up to the eighth dorsal vertebra. Hinged to either side of this are three metal bars

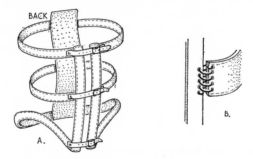

Fig. 10. McKee brace

passing respectively round the thorax, waist and pelvis. These three bars are joined together on each side at their anterior extremity by a vertically running bar. The metal is covered with soft leather and leather straps and buckles are attached to the front vertical bars at the level of the circumferential bands. There is no full length back lever, nor is there any apparatus for holding the shoulders back (*see* Fig. 10).

Attempts have been made to alter the position of hinging of the side bars. In particular, appliances have been made with a hinge in the centre of the top and bottom parts of the frame; this, in fact, is unsuitable since when the back frame is shaped to the lumbar curve, the hinge pins lose their alignment and it is impossible to open the appliance sufficiently for it to be put on. In fact, it has been found that closely fitting hinges between the back frame and each side bar are impracticable for the same reason. The simplest form of hinge is a short length of spiral spring, running through holes in both the back frame and the end of each side bar. This provides adequate fixation of the side bar to the frame but still allows play in the hinge so that curving of the back frame does not cause the hinges to bind.

The thoracic and waist bars are curved in one plane only to fit round the lower chest and waist at the level at which they arise from the back frame. The pelvic bar, however, rises slightly as it leaves the back frame, curves above the greater trochanters and then down again to the region of the body of the pubis. This allows clearance for the thighs when sitting, and also indicates to the patient which is the lower end of the frame.

Fitting

It is important to curve the posterior frame before fitting the side bars. This frame should fit the shape of the lumbar curve accurately and when it is in position it should be held there, the side bars being brought together in the front. It is helpful if the top line of the brace can approximate to a rectangle, the straight sides being posterior, anterior and lateral. This allows freedom in the posterior corners for movement of the posterior axillary folds, notably trapezius, and at the anterior corners freedom for the lower fibres of pectoralis major. The waist bars must be tight enough to support the appliance over the iliac crest and the pelvic bars should approximate in shape to the thoracic in that they have corners postero-laterally and antero-laterally. In this region, these corners allow free movement of the gluteal muscles and anteriorly freedom for muscles arising from the anterior superior iliac spine.

The anterior longitudinally running bars should be gently curved so that their upper extremity rests on the sternum and the lower extremity on the symphysis pubis. Between these two points the bars should fit comfortably against the abdominal wall. When applied in their correct position, the two vertical bars should be approximately 1 inch (2·5 cm) apart.

One advantage of this brace is that, as it has no fabric corset, the patient does not feel so hot and there is less constricting effect on the abdomen. It relies for its function purely on three-point pressure over the sternum, symphysis pubis and counter-pressure in the lumbar region.

GOLDTHWAIT SPINAL BRACE

This brace also consists of a shaped posterior frame with three encircling bars. It differs from the McKee brace, however, in that the encircling bars are rigidly fixed to the posterior frame

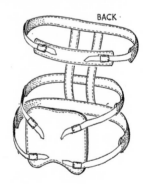

Fig. 11. Goldthwait brace

and extend some two-thirds of the circumference of the body only. The thoracic bar, which may reach high up into the axilla, ceases at the level of the anterior axillary folds and is completed by a leather strap and buckles. Lying on the abdomen is a leather pad suitably shaped and padded on its

deep aspect and four buckles on this receive straps arising from
the ends of the waist and pelvic bars (*see* Fig. 11).

In effect, this appliance works in a very similar manner to
that previously considered, but is more comfortable to wear in
that there is no longitudinally running bar and, because
the circumferential bars do not reach more than two thirds
of the way round the trunk, sitting is more comfortable. But
this movement involves a certain amount of flexion of the
lumbar spine and this implies that, not only is the sitting
posture more comfortable, but also, that the appliance is
slightly less efficient in maintaining a lumbar lordosis.

Because of the presence of the abdominal pad, there is some
compression of intra-abdominal contents but it is considerably
less marked than when a corset is worn.

ROBERT JONES BACKBRACE

Several variations of this appliance exist, some with
abdominal corsets. The essential feature is a broad pelvic band
made as an integral part of the back lever, which is shaped to
follow the spinal curves. Arising from the upper extremity of

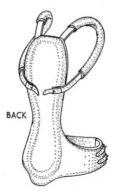

Fig. 12. Robert Jones brace

the back lever which reaches approximately to the level of the
third or fourth dorsal vertebra are two leather straps which
extend forward, one on each side, round the shoulders and

back through the axillae to be strapped on to the back lever (*see* Fig. 12).

When ordered for ladies, it is common to provide a fabric corset which underlies the pelvic band and extends round the abdomen from the level of the waist down to the gluteal folds. To this corset the suspenders are attached.

If the pelvic band is wide enough and carefully shaped to lie comfortably between the greater trochanters and the iliac crest, this appliance will give extremely good fixation to the pelvis but it is difficult to manufacture and fit a band of the width depicted which is still comfortable and does not produce localized bony pressure.

Many of these appliances are shown with groin straps but if fitting is accurate these should not be needed. The shape of the pelvic band and the curvature of the back lever fitting closely into the dorsal and lumbar spine should prevent the appliance from riding upwards, and this is the only function that groin straps have. If the appliance fits well, therefore, there is no necessity to supply these attachments.

TAYLOR BRACE

This appliance has a leather-covered metal framework consisting of a posterior rectangular frame, the side arms of which

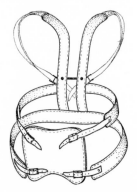

Fig. 13. Taylor brace

are extended up to the shoulders at the level of approximately the third dorsal vertebra. The pelvic bands extend two-thirds of the way round the trunk and are completed by a leather strap and buckle anteriorly. From the upward extension of the side bars, a leather strap passes across the shoulders and is buckled to the lower extremity of the dorsal bars. The waist bar on this model is replaced entirely by a fabric belt and buckle (*see* Fig. 13). It is common to supply this appliance also with perineal straps and the criticism given above holds good in this instance also. It can also be supplied with an abdominal pad to which is fixed the anterior extension of the pelvic band and the fabric waist strap. In this case, the appliance becomes very similar to a Goldthwait brace with the addition of shoulder straps.

FISHER JACKET

This brace, the use of which is normally restricted to severe scoliotics, consists of a stout posterior frame extending from the second sacral level up to perhaps the third or fourth dorsal vertebra and shaped to the patient's spine. From its lower extremity, two bars extend around the pelvis just above the greater trochanters and are completed at their anterior ends by a strap and buckle. Arising from the back lever, just above the pelvic bands, is a bar on either side, which curves above the iliac crest and descends to meet the pelvic band at its anterior extremity. Arising from the pelvic band at its mid-lateral point is a vertical bar on either side, which is connected to the iliac crest band and then continued up to the axilla. At its upper end it is joined to the upper part of the back lever by a horizontal bar and bears at its extreme upper limit a padded crutch piece which extends forwards to the anterior aspect of the shoulder. This metal framing is covered with leather and the space between the side bars and the back lever is filled in with fabric, usually incorporating some form of lacing device. Fabric frequently completes the anterior part of the pelvic support, filling in the space lying below the level of the umbilicus.

Extending from the anterior extremities of the crutch arm

pieces are fabric straps which ascend across the shoulder and pass down the back, crossing over at the junction of the mid and upper thirds of the back lever and extend round the opposite side to be buckled to the pelvic band of the contra-lateral side (*see* Fig. 14).

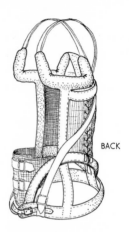

Fig. 14. Fisher jacket

Thus, when one of these appliances correctly fitted is applied, it gives firm support round the pelvis, the shoulders are held against the back lever by the crutch pieces and also by the shoulder straps and any tendency to scoliosis can be corrected by adjustment of the postero-lateral lacing. In addition, the abdomen is held firmly in by the abdominal corset and the appliance, therefore, can act as a correcting as well as support-ing brace.

The disadvantage of an appliance of this sort, apart from its weight, is great difficulty in fitting. The patient is usually grossly mis-shapen and very accurate adjustments and careful padding of the various bars are necessary. This type of appliance in theory could be expected to control the increasing kyphosis of an osteoporotic spine but, in fact, it is less efficient than one would expect. So long as the patient makes a conscious attempt to stand upright the corset will co-operate but the depressors of the pectoral girdle rapidly tire when he is constantly leaning forward in the appliance. The shoulders, therefore, are passively hunched by the crutch pieces and this allows the dorsal curve to increase.

The writer has not seen any adult, in full possession of his faculties, who is prepared to wear a brace of this nature as a corrective appliance. Children take to it remarkably rapidly but it is well recognized that children will ignore considerably greater discomfort than adults are prepared to accept. Also, of course, an appliance of this sort has not much scope for adjustment in size and frequent new braces are necessary when used for the growing child.

This sort of appliance is often accepted very readily by the patient who is mentally as well as physically disabled and it has been found the best method of treating the gross spinal deformities often seen associated with mental deficiency.

JEWETT BRACE

This appliance fulfils ideally the three-point pressure technique so well described by Charnley. It consists of two strips of aluminium curved in three planes, joined together anteriorly by pads which fit over the sternum and symphysis pubis. From the sternal pad the bar on each side passes laterally, skirts the anterior axillary fold, descends in the mid-lateral line to just below the level of the iliac crest and then curves forwards, skirting the fold of the groin, to join the symphyseal pad.

The third point of pressure is provided by a small rectangular frame in the lumbar region, from either corner of which a fabric strap passes to meet the mid-lateral bars already described, on either side (*see* Fig. 15).

This appliance restricts flexion of the lumbar spine by pressure in the three mechanically desirable places. It does little to control rotation, except for that limitation provided by the close fit of the mid-lateral parts of the bars.

Accurate fitting is essential in this appliance. The sternal pad, for example, is not vertical when the patient is standing but slopes downwards and forwards. This means that the upper extremity of the lateral bars must be twisted in their length to allow this slope, but must revert to a true sagittal line in the mid-lateral position.

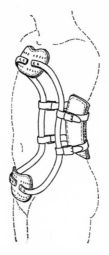

Fig. 15. Jewett brace

In addition, there is considerable tendency for this appliance to drop downwards when the patient is standing and this can only be prevented by carefully fitting the mid-lateral parts of the bars into the waist so that they sit on the iliac crests. If the bars do not reach the mid-lateral line exactly and the width of the bar does not lie in the sagittal plane, there is considerable danger of the anterior margin of this part of the bar producing localized pressure on the iliac crest, leading to skin necrosis in this region.

Having fitted this type of appliance carefully, the patient must be encouraged to walk, sit, stand, lie, walk again and then reassess the fit. It will probably only show the defects after wear for some hours and, therefore, it is advisable to arrange for adjustments to be made at frequent intervals during the first week or so.

One great advantage of this appliance is that there is no

abdominal corset whatsoever, no restriction to abdominal distension following meals and a great feeling of freedom for the patient. Corrective forces are applied over broad bone surfaces by relatively large pads in the areas which are most effective mechanically and many patients who have previously been supplied with appliances with encircling components have spoken favourably of the freedom which they notice when wearing a Jewett brace.

The important thing to note here is that the fit is much more critical than with most of the other appliances but if one is prepared to take the trouble to ensure close and accurate fitting, the final result is well worth it.

MOULDED APPLIANCES

LEATHER

A moulded leather brace made to a plaster cast and reinforced with metal bands at appropriate sites can be an extremely comfortable appliance to wear for the fixed scoliotic.

The difficulty is that moulded leatherwork is time consuming and requires the expert. Workers in this field are in extremely short supply and it is usually necessary for the supplier to subcontract the work out. This, in turn, involves delay, secondhand knowledge and difficulty with adjustments.

The appliance requires the making of a positive cast which is usually undertaken by the fitter who, when the cast is dry, passes it on to the craftsman. The positive can be adjusted to allow reduction or increase of pressure where necessary and the article made to the modified cast. Following the leatherwork and finishing, bracing with metal is applied to the outer surface, where indicated, and even after finishing some alteration in fit can be achieved by localized stretching of the leather and the use of softening agents or steam. Patients who have severe deformities and have used braces as previously described often welcome the provision of a moulded leather corset but, as in the previous example, fit is critical and difficult.

When assessing the adequacy of such an appliance, one must accept the deformity as it is and make no attempt to correct it. This appliance is made with the idea of providing support in an established position. Having accepted that position, one must allow room round the upper margin to enable the patient to carry out normal arm movements and similarly the lower margin must be cut away in the groins to enable the patient to sit in comfort.

The accurate fitting of the appliance will prevent it riding up or down when sitting.

PLASTIC CORSETS

Custom-made corsets in thermo-setting plastics have been available for some years and have proven very satisfactory in many instances. As with block leatherwork, they are made to a positive cast but may be made in two sections independently and buckled together on one or both sides (*see* Fig. 16).

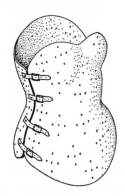

Fig. 16. Polythene corset

They have certain advantages over the block leatherwork in that although the provision of the positive cast requires the same degree of skill in either case, the manufacture of the polythene splint does not require the same craftsmanship. It can more easily be trimmed than the leather variety and the edges can be smoothed off with sandpaper, following which a hot iron is used to remove the residual roughness.

It is, however, less well ventilated than the leather brace and in spite of holes being drilled in many sites, patients frequently complain of sweating. Minor adjustments to the fit can be made by rubbing gently with a hot spoon which will produce localized stretching but localized shrinking is much more difficult to achieve.

TEMPORARY CORSETS

In recent years many temporary corsets have appeared on the market, the aim of which is to provide immediate support for the spine, until a definitive corset can be supplied (*see* Fig. 17).

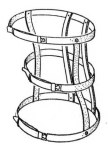

Fig. 17. Linflex spinal support

PLASTIC TEMPORARY CORSETS

The Wakeman type consists of a preformed anterior shell which comes in three sizes for males and three for females. The brace is completed by three plastic straps which pass round the back, fitting over studs borne on the margins of the anterior shell. These appliances are easy to clean after use and can be reissued as indicated.

Because of the provision of three sizes most people can be accommodated but this is not to say that they are fitted. The appliance is perfectly satisfactory as a temporary measure to control the patient's symptoms for a week or two until a definitive corset is supplied. The appliance is not, however, as comfortable as a plaster jacket although, of course, it takes far less time to apply.

FABRIC CORSETS

Many such corsets have been made, some with buckle fastenings and others with Velcro. The stiffeners used are usually of soft metal which can be readily shaped to approximate to the patient's trunk but there are a number available which have inserts of soft thermoplastic which are bent to an appropriate shape simply by being moulded against the patient's trunk when the anterior buckles are tightened (*see* Fig. 18).

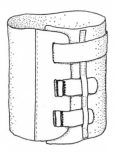

Fig. 18. Fabric corset

It is probable that the encircling corsets serve only to remind the patients to be careful of unguarded movements and to hold their backs straight. Certainly if a patient wearing one of these appliances tries to move it will offer little resistance.

It is difficult to see how, in view of the extremes of size, weight and girth met with in an Orthopaedic Clinic, any 'off the shelf' appliance can be expected to do more than provide an approximation to the definitive appliance. It is reasonable to provide these facilities if the patient's need for restriction and control is not great but one should bear in mind that their efficiency is considerably less than that of a custom-made appliance.

THERMOPLASTIC CORSETS MOULDED ON THE PATIENT

A brace cut from a sheet of polythene and lined with a layer of Polyurethane foam can be heated in an infra-red oven, applied when plastic to the patient and bandaged into position until cool. This is applied with the Polyurethane against the patient and the insulating effect of the air trapped within the foam prevents the patient from being burnt. Theoretically this provides an extremely good appliance but in practice it is difficult to get the corset apposed to the patient's skin rapidly enough and bandaged in position before it cools (*see* Fig. 19).

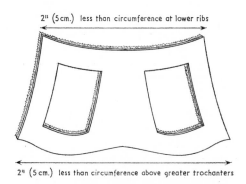

2" (5 cm.) less than circumference at lower ribs

2" (5 cm.) less than circumference above greater trochanters

Fig. 19. Pattern of thermoplastic corset

If a thermoplastic material is to be used, it is much more effective if a positive cast of the trunk is made, the appliance and the cast heated before the moulding takes place. This gives greater trim for accurate fitting of the appliance and the finished article can be worn with less discomfort than if it had been moulded direct to the patient. A further benefit gained is that the appliance, in fitting the trunk more closely, advertises its presence less through the clothes.

THREE

Upper Limb Appliances

NERVE INJURIES IN THE UPPER LIMB

For each nerve the picture varies according to several criteria:

(*a*) The level of the lesion determines which muscles are likely to be involved.

(*b*) The exact distribution of the nerve in each patient also has a marked effect. This is particularly so when the hand is considered, since nerve distribution in the hand shows a good deal of individual variation. Thus it is quite common for some of the thenar muscles to have supply from both the ulnar and median nerves, or to find a muscle, classically supplied by the median nerve, but having an ulnar supply in a particular case.

(*c*) The treatment the patient has received since the nerve injury occurred will have a great bearing on the mobility of the joints in the part affected. In those patients who have been exposed to long and continued splinting, the joints will be stiff and rigid with very little movement possible. These present a very different problem from those cases which have been encouraged to move the affected joints, even if this movement has been, by necessity, passive. In the latter event, the adhesions round the joint, and the fibrosis within the capsule, will be reduced to a minimum,

36

and the range of movement will probably approximate to a full normal excursion.

(d) Finally, the time that has elapsed since the date of the injury must be considered, particularly in conjunction with (c). The combination of these two aspects may give the surgeon a clue as to the likelihood of recovery of movement in any particular joint by active splinting.

One must also bear in mind the needs of the patient. It may well be that a patient is unable to carry out particular movements or actions under test conditions, but when trying to perform similar activities at home, or in his work, he may have found an alternative way of producing the same effect, or even accomplish it by a trick movement. The important consideration when dealing with patients with nerve injuries is that they should be able to carry out activities of normal daily living, together with those activities necessary in the course of their work, and it is of no great importance to the patient how these activities are carried out. If a particular trick movement enables a man to be financially independent and to carry out his normal job, then it is obvious that he should be allowed to continue with this trick movement, rather than spend a great deal of time attempting to persuade him to carry out the same activity in perhaps a less efficient manner.

For these reasons it is impossible to give hard and fast rules about which sort of splint should be used in which nerve inury. One can only give the overall pattern of splints available and indicate their advantages and disadvantages, leaving the surgeon concerned with the patient's treatment to decide on the best type of appliance, and perhaps to suggest suitable additions or modifications which may enable the appliance to be of more value to a given patient. So far as the hand is concerned, those factors which produce joint stiffness in any part of the body with splinting, are seen much more commonly. The main errors are in holding a joint in a position of strain, rather than one of function, and of obtaining immobilization by splinting for far too long.

The commonest positional errors seen in the upper limb are flexion of the wrist with the palm flat and the fingers straight. Care should also be taken to ensure that the thumb is held in a position of opposition rather than abduction, as is commonly found. The flexed position of the wrist is particularly troublesome, in that it produces stretching of the extensor muscles with subsequent increased tension in the tendons, producing hyperextension at the metacarpophalangeal joints. This in turn produces increased tension in the digital flexors, and the interphalangeal joints are pulled into a position of flexion. It is attention not only to the fit of the appliance, but also to the position in which the part is held which enables these errors to be avoided.

MEDIAN NERVE PARALYSIS

EFFECTS OF A HIGH LESION

The muscles affected here are pronator teres, flexor carpi radialis, flexor pollicis longus, pronator quadratus, flexor digitorum sublimis and the radial half of flexor digitorum profundus in the forearm. In the hand the abductor of the thumb, the opponens, and part of flexor pollicis brevis are denervated, resulting in wasting of the thenar eminence, and the thumb tends to lie in a plane parallel to the fingers. Opposition and abduction cannot be carried out in most cases, but in some people a small range of abduction can be achieved by use of the extensor muscles. The loss of pronation of the forearm and flexion of the wrist are rarely a problem, since these movements can be produced passively by gravity and the patient soon learns to relax the opposing muscles. The main practical problem, in fact, is loss of abduction and opposition of the thumb and most patients with a lesion of the median nerve, at whatever level, can carry out most tasks provided the thumb can be maintained in that position by a suitable appliance. There is a tendency for the metacarpophalangeal joints to the index and middle finger to go into slight hyperextension, but in practice this does not seem to cause a great deal of disability.

APPLIANCES AVAILABLE

(*a*) To overcome opponens paralysis:

(1) *Cholmeley's opponens splint.* This consists of a strip of Perspex or P.V.C. approximately $1\frac{1}{4}$ inches (3 cm.) wide which is carefully moulded to begin in the middle third of the palm, passing round the ulnar border of the palm, across the dorsum of the hand and back round the radial border to finish opposite the volar aspect of the first web. A tongue extending distally

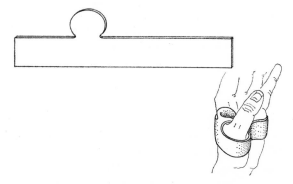

Fig. 20. Cholmeley's opponens splint

from this band passes through the first inter-digital cleft and is carefully moulded to fit into its concavity (*see* Fig. 20). This appliance effectively keeps the thumb in opposition, so that the digit is in the best position for function. The appliance must be very carefully shaped for the individual hand, and the stability of the appliance depends on its careful fitting in the first web. Indeed it must be very carefully shaped to lie immediately behind the bulge formed by the head of the second metacarpal on its palmar and radial aspects. It is this careful positioning, together with shaping of the flange passing round the thenar eminence which retains the appliance in position. There is no doubt that the appliance most effectively keeps the thumb in opposition, but the very closeness of the fit of the tongue in the first web produces some chafing of the skin at the level of the head of the second metacarpal, particularly if frequent flexion and extension movements of the second metacarpophalangeal joint are carried out.

(2) *Napier's opponens splint.* This consists of a wedge-shaped piece of sponge rubber covered with leather, which fits into the first cleft and prevents abduction of the thumb. It is held in position by two leather slings, one passing round the proximal

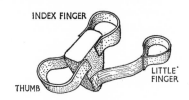

Fig. 21. Napier's opponens splint

phalanx of the thumb, and the other round the proximal phalanx of the index finger. The latter must be sufficiently loose to allow this sling to rotate round the index finger when the thumb is moved from flexion to extension. From the volar aspect of this wedge an elastic strap passes across the palm to terminate in a leather sling which is fitted round the proximal segment of the little finger. It is the presence of this elastic strap which tends to pull the little finger into opposition, and which maintains normal curvature of the metacarpal arch (*see* Fig. 21).

This appliance is more comfortable to wear for any length of time than the preceding one, but suffers from the disadvantage that the first interdigital cleft is largely occupied by the sponge rubber wedge. There is, too, a strong tendency for the little finger to be pulled across the palm, but if only fine work with the finger-tips is carried out, the appliance is generally very satisfactory.

(3) *Lively splint for median nerve paralysis.* This appliance consists of two lengths of plastic-covered spring wire which are

joined together at one end by a plastic trough, and at the other end by two parallel curved aluminium strips. The wires are so shaped that when the plastic trough is applied to the volar aspect of the neck of the proximal segment of the thumb, the shorter spring wire lies along the dorsal surface of the first web, and the longer spring curves round the volar aspect of the thenar eminence. The two parallel parts of the spring wires

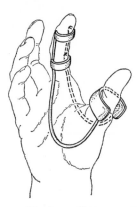

Fig. 22. Lively median nerve splint

then pass along either side of the index finger, the proximal aluminium strip lying at the level of the neck of the proximal phalanx and the distal sling on the volar aspect of the distal interphalangeal joint (*see* Fig. 22).

This appliance provides much more support than its appearance would suggest. The difficulties, however, are in the fit of the appliance. Very careful bending of the spring steels is necessary where they are attached to the plastic trough, in order to prevent the appliance steadily moving distally along the thumb and finally falling off. Similarly, careful fitting is needed at the index finger, and also to ensure that rotation of the splint on the index finger does not occur. Chafing of the skin has been noticed at the interphalangeal joint of the thumb, where a task involving a good deal of movement of this joint has been carried out for a lengthy period.

(4) Highet devised a very simple appliance, consisting of a

leather wrist strap and a small leather sling which is applied round the proximal phalanx of the thumb. These two are connected together by two lengths of elastic, which pass respectively to the radial and ulnar margins of the volar surface of the wrist strap. It is the relative tension in these two pieces of elastic which determines whether opposition or abduction are

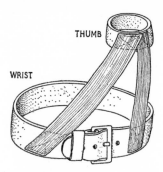

THUMB

WRIST

Fig. 23. Highet's median nerve splint

most favoured (*see* Fig. 23). In theory the appliance should be very satisfactory, but in practice one finds that if the elastic is too weak, the opposing muscles readily overcome it, and if it is strengthened, wrist flexion is produced. There is also frequently some difficulty in rotation of the wrist strap if the strip of elastic passing to the radial border is stronger than that to the ulnar side.

ULNAR NERVE PALSY

APPEARANCE

In a lesion of this nerve at or above the elbow, the forearm muscles involved are flexor carpi ulnaris, and the ulnar half of flexor digitorum profundus. In the hand there is loss of function of the hypothenar eminence and of adductor pollicis, together with most of the interossii and lumbricals. The hand therefore adopts the position of 'main-en-griffe' with hyperextension of the metacarpophalangeal joints and flexion of the interphalangeal joints. This clawing is much less marked on the index and middle fingers in most cases, since these lumbricals are usually supplied by the median nerve.

(1) *Passive supporting appliance.* The classic appliance used here is the rigid type of knuckleduster splint which consists of two strips of mild steel, each approximately an inch (2·5 cm.) wide. One is shaped to fit across the dorsal aspect of the proximal

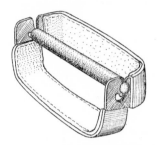

Fig. 24. Knuckleduster splint

phalanges of the four fingers and has a flange extending palmar-wards on either side, and the other adopts a similar position across the dorsal aspects of the necks of the four metacarpals. The flanges on each of these strips overlap opposite the volar aspects of the metacarpal heads, and are joined together by a rod which forms a hinge pin on each side of the hand. The metal strips are, of course, suitably padded and covered (*see* Fig. 24).

(2) *Active correcting appliance.* The above rigid type of knuckleduster has largely been replaced by the spring steel knuckleduster. This is made in two forms. In one pattern there are padded bars across the dorsal aspect of the metacarpals and the proximal phalanges, and these two are joined together by steel wire which is formed into a spring opposite the metacarpophalangeal joints. These springs are connected

across the palmar aspects of the metacarpophalangeal joints by a transverse bar (*see* Fig. 25).

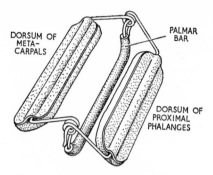

DORSUM OF
META-
CARPALS

PALMAR
BAR

DORSUM OF
PROXIMAL
PHALANGES

Fig. 25. Lively knuckleduster splint

In the second design, the dorsal pads are rigidly fixed together by a bent rod on the radial and ulnar borders of the metacarpals and a coiled spring passes from each of the four corners to the margins of the hand, level with the palm, and the palmar bar is fixed to the extremities of these four springs. The dorsal pads can swivel on the rods during movement of the metacarpophalangeal joints (*see* Fig. 26).

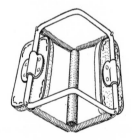

Fig. 26. Lively knuckleduster splint (another design)

A temporary appliance, described by Pruce, can be made very simply by use of a leather wrist strap, attached to which is a length of elastic terminating in a small leather sling which passes round the little and ring fingers. When the wrist strap is applied it is so positioned that the elastic lies on the palmar aspect of the fourth and fifth metacarpals, and this then pulls the fourth and fifth metacarpophalangeal joints into flexion. The appliance is very similar to the Highet splint used in an opponens paralysis, and suffers from the same disadvantages. Pruce states that this appliance has no value in the established deformity, but is helpful in that it prevents rigidity of the metacarpophalangeal joints developing (*see* Fig. 27).

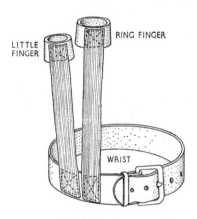

Fig. 27. Pruce's ulnar palsy splint

COMBINED MEDIAN AND ULNAR PALSY

This is a common combination seen in lesions of the upper limb, particularly when they have occurred in the region of the wrist. It produces great interference with the function of the hand, but it can to a considerable extent be diminished by use of Baker's modification of the lively knuckleduster splint. This consists of the lively knuckleduster splint mounted on which is a spring wire extending from the radial side of the dorsal plate over the metacarpals. This projects in a palmar direction and has on its end a plastic trough which bears against the ulnar border of the first metacarpal of the thumb, and acts as a stay to keep the thumb in abduction (*see* Fig. 28).

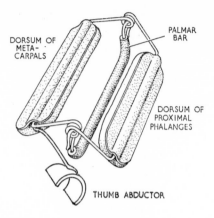

Fig. 28. Baker's modification of lively knuckleduster splint

RADIAL PALSY

DESCRIPTION

In a lesion of this nerve the extension of the elbow, wrist and fingers may be affected, depending on the level of the lesion. Extension of the elbow produces no practical problems in the great majority of cases, since it can be carried out by gravity. But, of course, the patient would be unable, in a high lesion, to extend the elbow when reaching up for something on a shelf.

As a secondary effect of wrist drop, there is usually weakness of grip, because there is relative lengthening of the digital flexors, and the tendon excursion is insufficient to produce full flexion of the digits into the palm with the wrist in this position. One often finds that, if the wrist can be held in a slightly dorsiflex position, the intrinsic muscles will extend the inter-phalangeal joints but the metacarpophalangeal joints still remain in the flexed position.

Elbow.   No appliances are necessary for maintaining extension of the elbow if the arm is used below shoulder level.

Wrist.   Passive supporting appliances.

A palmar slab made of any of the commonly used materials, i.e. plaster of Paris or any of the more rigid plastics, can, by maintaining the wrist in slight dorsiflexion, allow the fingers to be used with much greater ease. Similarly, many rigid splints are made from mild steel which is suitably bent to pass along the margins of the forearm, and is maintained by appropriately sited dorsal and volar straps.

Active wrist supports

Splints similar to that described immediately above can be made with a single spring turn on either side of the wrist, which does allow a small range of flexion to be carried out against the resistance of the spring. But this range is so small that it can, for practical purposes, be ignored. When the wrist is held in dorsiflexion, the course of the flexor tendons is lengthened, and therefore the metacarpophalangeal joints are pulled into more flexion than when wrist is allowed to hang down (*see* Fig. 29).

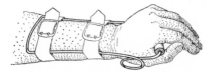

Fig. 29. Lively cock-up splint

FINGERS

The main problem with use of an appliance with radial palsy is to ensure that the fingers can be used to their best advantage, and it is to this end that most of the appliances in use today have been designed.

47

PASSIVE SUPPORTING APPLIANCE

The simplest solution is to produce a palmar slab which extends to the level of the necks of the proximal phalanges, and this, by supporting the metacarpophalangeal joints, does allow the intrinsic muscles to extend the interphalangeal joints and the digital flexors to carry out their normal function. This appliance is used with part of it encircling the thumb to maintain it in extension and opposition, thus putting the hand in the best position of function. The appliance has the appearance of a scaphoid plaster.

ACTIVE SPLINTS

These appliances have in common a chassis which is fixed to the forearm and dorsal aspect of metacarpal region to carry spring-loaded supports for the digits. They come in many forms, and there is little to choose between them except in a few cases where special requirements must be met:

(a) *The Brian Thomas splint* consists of a dorsal forearm slab, sometimes extended to cover the metacarpal region. From this extends forward a strong curved spring steel, which carries on its end a transverse bar. The spring steel passes through the cleft between the middle and ring fingers, and

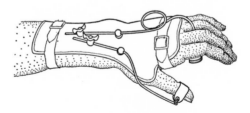

Fig. 30. Brian Thomas splint

the transverse bar lies on the volar aspect of the proximal phalanges of the four fingers. It produces a simultaneous extension of the metacarpal phalangeal joints of these digits. It may also bear a separate spring, carrying on its extremity a leather sling, to produce extension of the carpometacarpal and metacarpophalangeal joints of the thumb (*see* Fig. 30).

A refinement of this splint consists of making the forearm and metacarpal portions of the dorsal slab separately, joined together by a spring controlled hinge, so that movements of the wrist can take place without movements of the fingers. The appliance produces good extension of the wrist, but suffers from the disadvantage that individual finger movements cannot be carried out with any ease.

(b) *Lloyd's deviation hand splint* is a similar appliance except that the dorsal spring carrying the bar for finger extension is mounted on a swivel over the level of the wrist joint, and

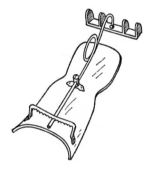

Fig. 31. Lloyd's deviation hand splint

the spring is extended to a serrated bar at the proximal end of the dorsal slab. Thus movements of the proximal end of the spring across the serrated bar produce radial or ulnar deviation of the wrist at the other end of the appliance. This may be of some value when one is faced with a partial radial palsy only, or perhaps when it is combined with injury to another nerve in the forearm (*see* Fig. 31).

(c) To avoid the disadvantage of the Brian Thomas appliance where individual finger movement is restricted, many varieties of splint have been made which have support for each individual finger. These consist of a fixed aluminium or plastic dorsal slab, or of wire splints of the cockup variety which extend from the proximal third of the forearm to the necks of the metacarpals and placed across their distal aspect is a series of four studs, each of which carries a small coiled spring passing forward along the line of the fingers and having on their extremities small leather or wire loops to support each digit in turn. By suitable variation of the strength of the wire supporting the digits, one can balance the flexors of the fingers with a good deal of precision (*see* Fig. 32).

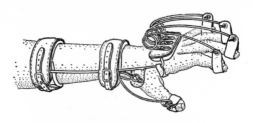

Fig. 32. Exeter radial palsy splint

Other splints based on the same principle have been used which consist of a plastic dorsal slab being bent up at right angles at the distal end at the level of the metacarpal necks. These carry elastic strips passing from their proximal end through holes in the right-angled portion and again terminating in slings round the proximal phalanges (*see* Fig. 33).

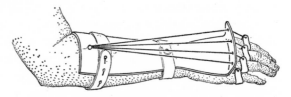

Fig. 33. Plastic radial palsy splint

These appliances undoubtedly produce extension of the metacarpophalangeal joints but there is a strong tendency for hyperextension to be produced. There is also a good deal of difficulty in preventing rotation of the splint round the forearm since the asymmetrical pull on the thumb cannot be counterbalanced.

(*d*) To avoid the need for such large appliances the *Bristow traction glove* was devised. This initially consisted of a simple glove which bore on its dorsal surfaces spring steels passing along the length of each metacarpal and along the appropriate finger. It was found during use, however, that a great deal of pressure was applied to the skin over the heads of the metacarpals during flexion of the digits, and to avoid this and to make the forces of extension more effective, the spring steels were replaced by elastic straps which passed over sponge rubber bolsters lying on the dorsal aspect of the metacarpal necks.

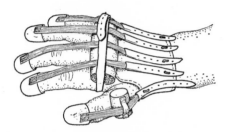

Fig. 34. Bristow traction glove

Later, most of the glove was dispensed with, and the elastic straps terminated in soft leather thimbles. As with the full glove this type suffers from the great disadvantage that tactile sensibility is greatly diminished when the appliance is in use. It is very useful, of course, if the patient is able to do his job under direct vision, but for anything else he is at a disadvantage and is probably better off not wearing the appliance (*see* Fig. 34).

(*e*) A recent innovation has been the use of spring steel appliances combined with plastic troughs to support the digits. One such 'Spider splint' for use in radial palsy consists of four lengths of spring steel covered with plastic tubing. These radiate from a plastic trough which is worn on the volar aspect of the proximal phalanx of the thumb and the four steels pass across the dorsum of the hand on the ulnar side of each of the fingers and each terminates in a plastic trough, which supports the intermediate phalanx of the appropriate digit (*see* Fig. 35).

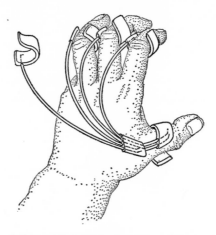

Fig. 35. Spider splint (little finger trough not yet in place)

This appliance does nothing to overcome the wrist drop, but it does produce a surprisingly large amount of extension of the thumb and fingers. It has the advantage that parts of the fingers are left free and there is no interference of sensibility in this area. The appliance does, however, suffer from the disadvantage that fitting is extremely critical, and very often one finds that the wearer spends as much time concentrating on maintaining the appliance in position, as he does in using his hands. It provides much more power than one would expect, however, and if one has an intelligent patient who can co-operate with the fitting, and describe his difficulties in detail, the appliance can be extremely effective. In some cases, its use with a simple cockup splint has produced an even greater improvement in function.

FINGER SPLINTS

The greatest difficulty found in splinting the digits is maintaining the appliance in position, particularly if the splint is to have any 'lively' function.

MALLET FINGER

The difficulty in maintaining an appliance in position with this deformity has led to many ingenious devices being described. Only two are in common use at the present time and each of these appears to be no more satisfactory than a well-moulded skin-tight plaster.

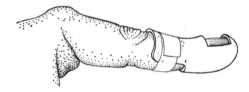

Fig. 36. Mallet finger splint

The earliest of these designs to appear was the polythene mallet-finger splint, which consists of a preformed short cylinder of polythene with a cut-out for the finger-nail and a tongue extending proximally on the dorsal surface of the intermediate phalanx. Having chosen the correct size and applied it, it is maintained in position by strapping passed round the proximal end. It will, if correctly applied and maintained, hold the terminal interphalangeal joint at full extension, but it does ensure that the digit is little used (*see* Fig. 36).

The more recently described 'frog' plaster, preformed in

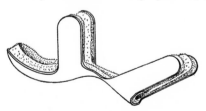

Fig. 37. Frog splint

aluminium and lined with foam rubber, is as effective as the above appliance, but a little more cumbersome to wear (*see* Fig. 37).

FINGER DEVIATION SPLINT

This appliance has been described for correction of deviation of the distal phalanx in cases of arthritis deformans. It consists of a single turn of wire passing from the ulnar side of the tip of the finger, across the volar aspect to the radial side of the proximal phalangeal joint, and then continuing across the dorsum of the finger to the ulnar side of the proximal phalanx. There are small pads at the margins of the digit protecting the

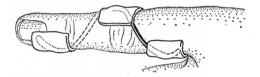

Fig. 38. Finger deviation splint

points at which pressure is applied. The splint does allow a small range of extension and flexion of the finger but one usually finds that the patient uses other digits in preference to the one under the influence of the splint. Correction is only available while the splint is in position, and it must not be assumed that a cure of the deformity will result (*see* Fig. 38).

FLEXION CONTRACTURE SPLINTS

The use of splints in this category depends on the digit being fixed in flexion with lack of extension, and all appliances therefore maintain a steady extension force on the digits, with the aim of stretching the tight structures, and thus increasing the range of extension.

(a) *Dupuytren's contracture splint*. This appliance consists of an appropriate number of segments of a Bristow's extension glove. Thus if a single digit is involved in Dupuytren's contracture then one ray of the glove can be used.

(b) *The safety-pin finger extension splint.* This consists of lateral spring wires connected across the volar surface of the proximal and distal segments of the finger and across the dorsal surface of the intermediate, by small leather-covered

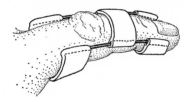

Fig. 39. Safety-pin extension splint

troughs. The lateral springs are appropriately bent to maintain a constant extension strain on the affected interphalangeal joints. The appliance is very simple, and can be readily made, but once the position of the digit approximates to full extension, there is considerable difficulty in maintaining the appliance in place (*see* Fig. 39).

(c) *Armchair finger extension splint.* This consists of a pad under the volar surface of the metacarpal head, and from it pass lateral wires turned into three coils at the level of the proximal phalanx. Extending further forward than these

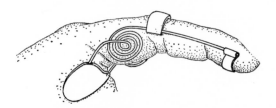

Fig. 40. Armchair extension splint

coils are side arms which are joined together across the pulp of the finger by a small metal trough. The extension force of these two coil springs provides the correcting force on the contracted digit, and counter-pressure is applied by a metal trough extending across the dorsal aspect of the proximal interphalangeal joint from one coil spring to the other (*see* Fig. 40).

This appliance provides a better corrective force than does either of the two appliances mentioned above, and in addition, allows a much greater range of movement of the digit while held in the splint. It also stays in position much more readily than do other appliances already mentioned.

(*d*) *Finger flexion splint.* This appliance consists of three pads which lie on the dorsal aspect of the three segments of the affected finger. These pads consist of a curved metal plate

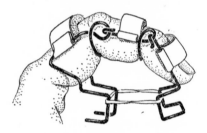

Fig. 41. Finger flexion splint

lined on the surface in contact with the digit by a small piece of sponge or similar soft material. The pads are coupled together by wire loops which also pass across the volar aspect of the interphalangeal joints. Projecting in a palmar direction from the proximal corners of the pad on the proximal phalanx and from the distal corners of the pad on the distal phalanx are four stiff wires which, in use, are pulled together by an elastic band (*see* Fig. 41). Thus the finger is under constant flexion strain by the elastic bands and the amount of flexion strain can be varied by alteration of the size of elastic band chosen and also by bending the side arms.

It is a very satisfactory appliance so far as flexing the digit is concerned, but the projecting wires on the volar surface of the finger do interfere with closure of the hand,

and with function of the other digits. If the patient can carry out one-handed tasks, the appliance is very satisfactory for the other hand, but he will find great difficulty in using a knife and fork, putting his hand in his pocket, and in carrying out many other simple daily tasks.

SHOULDER ABDUCTION SPLINT

Several types of splint have been devised for this purpose, the difficulty always being to provide suitable purchase on the trunk to support the weight of the arm, and also to preform an appliance which is sufficiently adjustable to fit most people. At one time it was considered that all ruptures of the rotator cuff should be treated with the arm in abduction, thus relaxing the torn muscles, and approximating muscle insertion to origin. In addition, many fractures of the upper part of the humerus were treated in this way, but in recent years it has become customary to support the limb in a sling, when in previous times abduction was considered essential.

One of the earliest abduction splints consisted of metal troughs, one half encircling the pelvis and the other half encircling the thorax. These are fixed together by a single vertical bar in the mid-axillary line, to the top of which was hinged a trough to accommodate the arm, and hinged to that, a trough to accommodate the forearm, terminating in a ball pad in the palm, producing a small degree of cockup. Passing

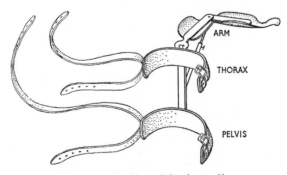

Fig. 42. Shoulder abduction splint

57

from the lower part of the vertical bar to the elbow was an oblique strut, which had some form of adjustment on it to vary the degree of abduction. It was customary too, for the hinge at the axillary end of the vertical bar to have some means of adjustment for flexion of the shoulder joint (*see* Fig. 42).

This appliance is held in position by straps passing round the pelvis just below the iliac crests and also round the thorax. It is usually necessary too, to have an oblique strap passing from the pelvic trough across the opposite shoulder. The upper limb is simply bandaged in position in its support.

The appliance does carry out the task set for it satisfactorily, but it is a very heavy appliance, cumbersome to wear, difficult to adjust, difficult to wear under clothes and impossible to apply over the clothes.

For this reason many simpler varieties have been produced, most of them based on the bent wire principle.

THE LITTLER-JONES ARM ABDUCTION SPLINT

This consists of rigid round rods, shaped to half encircle the pelvis, to pass vertically up the front and back of the thorax, and then bent at right angles to continue down the arm. The bars carry leather slings, passing from one to the other, which

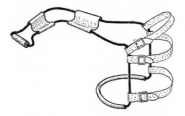

Fig. 43. Littler-Jones abduction splint

provide support for the upper limb, and at the hand it is customary to have a transverse wooden roller which can be gripped by the patient. The appliance is held on by two straps passing round the trunk and one passing round the opposite shoulder (*see* Fig. 43).

CANTILEVER SPLINT

In both the above appliances there is a great tendency for that part of the appliance attached to the trunk to slide distally and thus the abduction to steadily diminish throughout the day.

In an attempt to overcome this, Jordan described an abduction splint on a cantilever principle. This consists of two metal bars, passing from the shoulder on the uninjured side across the front and back of the chest, down either side of the arm and then at right angles to continue along the dorsal and volar aspects of the forearm. The bar on the dorsal aspect finishes at the level of the wrist, that on the volar surface being continued for another 3 inches (7·5 cm.) or so, and terminating in a hand grip. In the distal third of the forearm, these two bars are joined together by a metal trough, and at the level of the arm a leather sling passes between the two. Over the dorsal aspect of the affected shoulder a metal trough unites the two bars and this is well padded. At the other extremity of this splint where lies the uninjured shoulder, a metal trough passes through the uninjured axilla, and this too is well padded. It will be noted that when this splint is worn the upper arm is externally rotated on the shoulder; thus when the patient is standing up, the forearm is pointing towards the ceiling. With the splint in position, therefore, the arm tends to drop down to the side, and the sling takes the weight of the limb. The trough over the affected shoulder becomes the pivot and the end of the splint in the region of the contralateral axilla tends to rise but is held down by the weight of the contralateral arm.

Jordan states that this appliance can be pre-made, is readily adjustable and does not produce pressure on the iliac crest. The idea is most ingenious but it is obvious that the weight of the limb is being applied to the leather sling and to the hand grip approximately 15 inches (38 cm.) or 16 inches (40 cm.) from the metal trough over the affected shoulder, which forms the fulcrum. But the counter-balancing force is being applied some 10 inches (25 cm.) from the fulcrum. Obviously these two weights, although no doubt equal in the patient, are not satisfactorily balanced because of unequal leverage. One sees, therefore, that the splint on the affected side does tend to droop, and the contralateral shoulder becomes elevated. The patient

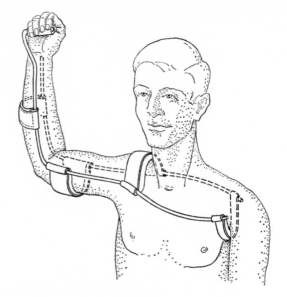

Fig. 44. Jordan's cantilever abduction splint

finds pressure on both the anterior and posterior axillary folds of the contralateral shoulder produces rubbing of the skin and a good deal of discomfort. There is no doubt, however, that the other attributes claimed by Jordan are correct.

ULNAR DEVIATION SPLINT

(a) SNAKE BANGLE

This appliance, made as a wide coil of either a thermoplastic material or in stout spring wire, has been used to control the ulnar deviation of rheumatoid disease. It should be considered a passive supporting appliance, rather than an active splint (*see* Fig. 45).

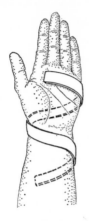

Fig. 45. Snake bangle

(*b*) ULNAR DEVIATION SPLINT

A lively ulnar deviation splint, has, however, been devised which consists of a metal frame passing along the dorsal aspect of the first web and extending across the metacarpal necks. An

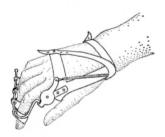

Fig. 46. Lively ulnar deviation splint

elastic strap completes the frame across the volar surface of the palm and across the wrist. Hinged to the distal end of the plate at the level of the second metacarpophalangeal joint is a small lever, bearing on its distal end a wire which passes across the dorsal aspects of the distal interphalangeal joints, and carrying slings which pass round each finger. At the proximal end of the lever a spring passes to the wrist strap. It is this which provides the correcting force. Again, this would seem to be a lively splint but in practice it acts as a passive correcting appliance, and, although movement is possible, this is not to be considered as treating the basic defect (*see* Fig. 46).

ELBOW SPLINTS

These appliances range from the simplest posterior gutter splint, made in one piece, to the more sophisticated hinged appliances. If all that is required is simple fixation of the elbow in a position of function and stability, the plastic posterior splint is usually sufficient. But if slightly heavier work is required it could be that a thermoplastic appliance almost

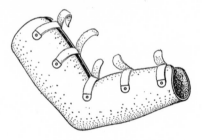

Fig. 47. Polythene elbow splint

completely encircling the arm, and held with straps and buckles, or Velcro, may be obligatory (*see* Fig. 47).

If movement is required while in this splint, of course, this presupposes encircling sections of the splint above and below the elbow, held together by distance pieces bearing hinges. In the absence of satisfactory muscle control, e.g. musculo-cutaneous palsy, it would be advisable to have these hinges with an automatic locking device incorporated, such as is used in artificial arms (*see* Fig. 48).

The wearer would have perhaps a choice of three positions of flexion, extension being achieved by exceeding the most flexed position, and the automatic release then allows the limb to drop into full extension. Each position of flexion then has to be achieved successively from that point. Once the elbow is in some degree of flexion its position prevents the splint falling off and prevents it from rotating on the arm. If the arm is held in full extension, however, it is impossible to retain the splint in position unless some sort of shoulder harness is used. This

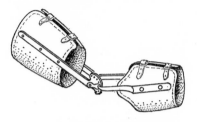

Fig. 48. Hinged elbow splint

the patient will undoubtedly find irksome. It is usually simpler for the patient to have the splint adjusted to its maximum degree of extension short of 180°, and it is common for the patient to wear the splint at this angle until a greater degree of flexion is required.

This appliance is particularly useful for a patient with a flail elbow but some retention of hand function.

FOUR

Abnormalities of the Lower Limb

APPLIANCES FOR CONGENITAL DISLOCATION OF THE HIP

These appliances are all based on the assumption that a dislocated hip, once reduced, will remain stable so long as that hip is kept in abduction. Since it is impossible to maintain one hip in full abduction without a comparable position on the other side, the appliances are all symmetrical and control the position of both femora.

DIVARICATOR

One of the earliest devices used was described by Putti and was termed a divaricator. It consists of three strips of wood

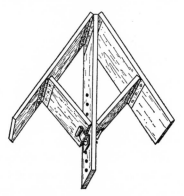

Fig. 49. Hip divaricator

64

approximately 15 inches (38 cm.) × 3 inches (7·5 cm.) hinged together at one end. The outer pieces of wood carried near their free ends a further hinged piece, the end of which, when abutted against the central strip, produced divarication of the outer sections. This appliance was placed between the abducted lower limbs of children, having first reduced the dislocation, and the limbs were bandaged in position. It had the advantage that the degree of abduction could be controlled, but the disadvantage that the appliance was not convenient for use unless the child was confined to bed (*see* Fig. 49).

THIGH ABDUCTION SPLINTS

Several patterns of this appliance based on the same principle have been described, the main difference being in the method of fixation to the trunk. The basic pattern consists of two thigh corsets made from block leather, plastic or some other firm material. These corsets lie with their central axes in the same straight line and are held apart by a bar of metal which is curved

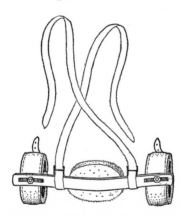

Fig. 50. Thigh abduction splint

to fit across the lower part of the trunk. Some authors have considered that the bar should lie across the pubis, whereas others have described it lying across the sacrum. It is clear that if it is applied lying across the sacrum it could rotate to lie

65

either caudally or over the pubic site unless some form of restriction is provided. This may consist either of a waist band and suspensory straps or the full shoulder harness. If applied across the pubis attempted adduction of the hips will allow the crossbar to move away from the body and pressure will be applied on the outer margins of the thigh corsets, producing redness and soreness of the skin just above the medial femoral condyles. Nevertheless, the anterior piece is generally more comfortable for the baby since he is able to lie on his back without undue pressure on the sacrum (*see* Fig. 50).

When the crossbar is in the dorsal position the pressure in attempted adduction tends to be more widely spread over the medial surfaces of the thighs and this does not lead to skin trauma, but unless the posterior bar is well padded, discomfort is found over the sacrum when the child is supine. Few children are willing to lie on their faces for most of the day.

THE BLANCHE SPLINT

This is a version of the above which consists of a central metal bar carrying a curved metal strip which, together with a fabric strap, encircles the waist. Hinged on either end of this bar and held with winged nuts is a short metal bar which carries on its free end the thigh corset. The corsets are fixed in such a way that their central axes can be adjusted. This appliance, there-fore, does allow the degree of flexion of the abducted hip to be adjusted to suit the needs of the particular case (*see* Fig. 51).

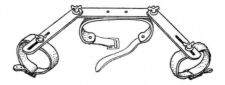

Fig. 51. Blanche splint

THE VON ROSEN SPLINT

This appliance consists of an H-shaped piece of malleable metal covered with a rubber compound. The crossbar of the

H is extended on either side. This appliance is very useful for maintaining flexion and abduction of the hip in small babies. In use the appliance is flattened, the baby placed on top and the upper extremities of the H carried down over the child's shoulders. The extended crossbar is then bent to lie round the waist. The hips are then reduced and the lower extremities of the H curved in a spiral round the thighs to hold them flexed and abducted at 90° each (*see* Fig. 52).

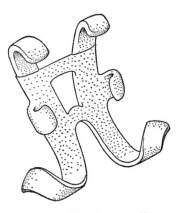

Fig. 52. Von Rosen splint

This appliance is very useful for the small baby but depends entirely on the child's muscles being unable to overcome the resistance of the metal frame. Thus it is unsuitable for a child who is gaining muscle strength where it is not possible to maintain the hips in the fully abducted and flexed position. Even a young baby can produce remarkable power of extension of the hips unless they are held in the fully flexed position.

FREJKA PILLOW

This appliance differs from those mentioned above in its design, but nevertheless fulfils the same function. It consists of a firm pillow, often divided transversely into three sections. It is applied to lie over the sacrum, between the legs and on to the abdomen. The width of the pillow should be just less than the distance between the popliteal fossae when the hips are flexed and abducted to 90°. The appliance is held in position by shoulder straps which should be joined together over the upper part of the dorsal region to prevent them sliding off the shoulders. Further straps pass from the lateral margin of the dorsal segment to a corresponding site on the ventral aspect, thus ensuring that the pillow is firmly held against the perineum (*see* Fig. 53).

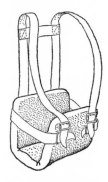

Fig. 53. Frejka pillow

SUMMARY

I think it is fair to say that the von Rosen and Frejka appliances are extremely useful in the young baby but are of little value in the older child. The abduction splints described in the earlier part of this chapter are, on the other hand, of more value for a child who is a few months old or who has needed either surgery or a prolonged time in a frog plaster. They could also be conveniently used as night splints in the final stages of treatment.

THE SHORT LEG

The classical examination for inequality of leg length takes place with the patient lying supine. The lower limbs are adjusted so that a line joining the anterior superior iliac spines is at right angles to the mid-line of the body. The distance from one anterior superior iliac spine to a bony prominence, usually the medial malleolus, is measured on one side and compared with the similar measurement of the other side. It is notoriously difficult to achieve an accurate reading and the method is quite inadequate for careful estimation when considering the degree of raise to be added to a patient's shoe.

Indeed, since inequality of leg length is quite unimportant when the patient is lying down, the most accurate, practical method of measurement is as follows. The patient should stand, taking equal weight on both feet, the knees to be straight and the pelvis tilted if this is necessary to get both feet on the floor. The distance from the anterior superior iliac spine to the floor is then measured and the difference between the two sides will indicate the amount of shortening. Should the position detailed above be impossible to achieve, the short leg is supported on wooden blocks until this condition can be achieved. Measurement of both sides is then made and to the difference between these two sides is added the height of the wooden blocks to give an accurate measurement of the total difference.

When considering how best to compensate for this shortening by alterations of footwear, one must take into account several features, notably the degree of shortening which is present, how much of this can be safely compensated by tilting the pelvis, how much the raise necessary can be compensated by leaving the foot in equinus and how much of the footwear can be hidden by the patient's clothes. It is obvious that a raise of 1 inch (2·5 cm.) would be clearly seen in the shoes of a young woman but would largely be hidden by a man's trousers.

Also, a shortening of 1½ inches (3·8 cm.) could be achieved by adapting a man's shoe, whereas a similar shortening in a woman would require a custom-made shoe.

There is commonly an inequality of leg-length in the normal individual and differences up to ½ inch (1·25 cm.) can be readily ignored. Beyond this, some degree of correction is advisable because the pelvic tilting of the uncorrected state leads to a scoliosis which, in the long run, will predispose towards lumbar degenerative changes, backache and subsequent morbidity.

(1) Raises up to $\frac{3}{8}$ inch (1 cm.) (i.e. $\frac{7}{8}$ inch (2·2 cm.) total shortening, $\frac{1}{2}$ inch (1·25 cm.) of which is uncorrected) can be achieved by insertion of a cork or leather wedge to the inner aspect of the heel of the shoe. No alteration to the shoe itself is required, beyond sticking this wedge in place; therefore, one wedge will be needed for each pair of shoes.

(2) Raises in excess of this amount and up to 1 inch (2·5 cm.) in height, can be accommodated in a man's shoe by addition to the heel, with perhaps a little reduction of the other heel. When these raises are inserted, it is necessary that the posterior

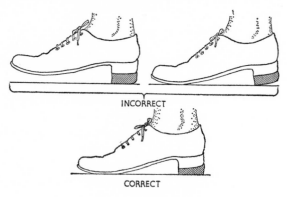

INCORRECT

CORRECT

Fig. 54. Heel raise

edge of the heel should be raised to a greater extent than the leading edge. If this obliquity of the heel is not produced, the patient will stand either with the leading edge of the heel and the sole of the shoe on the ground, or with the plantar surface of the heel on the ground and the sole clear. While the necessity for this wedging is apparent to surgical shoe-makers, it is often difficult to persuade the patient's local shoe-repairer to give a raise in this manner and an explanation to the patient is necessary in order that he may pass on the information. The amount of raise necessary is applied at the posterior edge of the heel and the raise of the anterior edge is estimated so that the flat of the heel and the sole of the shoe are on the ground at the same time. This wedge effect is best applied several layers below the surface of the heel in order that subsequent repairs of the shoe should not involve skiving layers of leather on each occasion repairs are performed (*see* Fig. 54).

(3) *Rand cork raise.* Raises of between 1 inch (2·5 cm.) and 3 inches (7·5 cm.) can be inserted in a commercial shoe by use of the Rand cork method. In this technique, the upper and the sole are separated and a cork block suitably shaped and covered

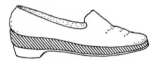

Fig. 55. Rand cork raise

with leather is inserted between the two. It is customary for this to have its maximum height posteriorly and to taper off towards the toe, thus the equinus position of the foot reduces the amount of cork necessary and, therefore, reduces the weight of the finished shoe. When ordering appliances of this nature, it is usual to stipulate the height at the heel and at the toe. Thus, a suitable order might read: 'Rand cork raise 2 inches (5 cm.) at the heel, tapering to ½ inch (1·25 cm.) at the toe' (*see* Fig. 55).

In recent years there has been an increasing number of shoes on the market in which the uppers and synthetic soles are welded together; a Rand cork cannot be applied to this variety of footwear.

(4) *Inner cork raise.* An increase of a similar height can be achieved by a surgical shoe with an inside cork block; thus a shoe is made of an orthodox design but with the upper deep

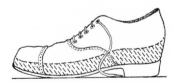

Fig. 56. Inner cork raise

enough to accommodate the patient's foot plus a cork block to compensate for his shortening. When ordering a raise of this type, it is essential to order a normal shoe for the other side. An appliance of this nature is obviously much less apparent when worn by a man, since only the lower part of the upper is seen below the trousers (*see* Fig. 56).

(5) *Outside cork compensator.* For raises of over $2\frac{1}{2}$ inches (6·25 cm.), an outside cork compensator can be used. This consists of an orthodox upper attached to a cork block of any height desirable. When the heel and sole are more than some 3 inches (7·5 cm.) in height, it is necessary to fit a bridge passing from the heel to the sole since this considerably strengthens the appliance. The appearance, however, is cumbersome and the weight considerable (*see* Fig. 57).

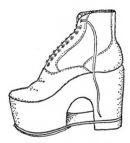

Fig. 57. Outside cork compensator

(6) *O'Connor boot.* For really large inequalities, the O'Connor boot is the most cosmetically acceptable. This consists of the upper of a shoe with the foot in considerable equinus. Extending from this is a light wooden strut covered with leather and shaped to fit into a shoe at the lower end. Thus inequalities in excess of 6 inches (15 cm.) can be adjusted and certainly in long trousers the appearance is of two normal feet. The difficulty, of course, is the considerable weight of these appliances, and also the great equinus in which the foot is placed resulting in the toes becoming cramped in the equinus boot. This can be corrected to some extent by very careful shaping of the boot

and by tight lacing, which brings its own problems (*see* Fig. 58).

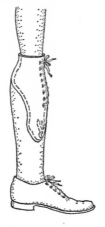

Fig. 58. O'Connor boot

FOOT-DROP

Aetiology. Two basic groups of conditions apply to foot-drop:

(*a*) paralysis of the muscles of the anterior compartment of the foot from any cause. Thus, anterior poliomyelitis, nerve lesions, etc., may be implicated.

(*b*) division of the extensor tendons.

In either group of conditions one is left with a simple foot-drop which is maintained by gravity. Some degree of inversion is frequently present, since the causative lesion often involves peroneal tendons also.

On examination, the position of the foot is distinctive; there is loss of function in the appropriate muscles and in cases of nerve injury or dysfunction, there may well be sensory disturbances also. The gait of the patient is pathognomonic, the leg on the affected side being excessively flexed at the hip and knee to allow the toe to clear the ground when taking a pace forward. When the foot is applied to the ground, the toe often

73

strikes the ground first and this produces a distinctive sound which can be recognized before the patient comes into view.

APPLIANCES

These consists of two varieties,
(*a*) passive prevention of the deformity and
(*b*) active correction of the deformity, the latter inevitably involving the use of springs of one sort or another.

Passive appliances. These consist of single or double irons, the decision between the two being made on the need to correct

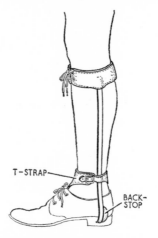

Fig. 59. Outside iron with inside T-strap and back-stop

inversion of the foot at the same time. In a foot-drop without varus, a single iron, usually outside to avoid trauma to the other leg, is provided. This is attached to the leg at the upper extremity by a calf band, and at its lower end a round spur articulates with a round socket set in the heel of the shoe. Attached to this socket is a short metal bar projecting laterally and proximally beside the heel which butts against the lower posterior 1 inch (2·5 cm.) of the iron and prevents the foot from falling into equinus. A strap passing closely round the ankle and the iron prevents the spur from sliding out of the socket during walking (*see* Fig. 59).

If inversion is also present, it may be controlled in a light person by an inside iron and outside T strap which also replaces the ankle strap, but in a heavy or very active patient double below-knee irons may be required, although a single back-stop is sufficient.

Because of the absolute bar to plantar flexion, the patient does experience difficulty when on stairs or when descending hills. On the stairs he is unable to plantarflex his foot to allow his toe to reach the tread below when descending, and on hills, when his heel strikes the ground, plantar flexion is unable to occur because of the back-stop. This means that the calf band is pressed firmly against the upper third of his leg by the influence of body weight and this, in turn, tends to produce early flexion of the knee. This is not a disadvantage in a patient who has a lateral popliteal nerve injury and normal quadriceps, but in a patient who suffers from the effects of anterior poliomyelitis and who may well have weak quadriceps, 'knee-shoot' may occur and lead to frequent falls.

ACTIVE CORRECTING APPLIANCES

(a) *Toe-raising spring*

A calf band is applied above the maximum circumference of the leg, to which is attached a Y-shaped leather strap carrying on the distal end a spiral spring. This passes to a D ring attached to the toecap of the shoe. It is usual to include a buckle to allow adjustment of length and tension (*see* Fig. 60).

The appliance possesses several disadvantages:

(1) It is unsightly, especially in females.
(2) The calf band, unless tightly strapped, is pulled down the leg.
(3) The spring causes wear on trousers.
(4) Deformity of the shoe at the level of the metacarpo-

phalangeal joint occurs and leads to a similar deformity of the foot.

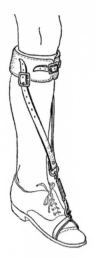

Fig. 60. Toe-raising spring

(b) *Side steel and spring*

An outside iron with a calf band has a hinge joint at the level of the ankle. The section below the hinge bears a projection forwards to which is attached a spiral spring stretched proximally via a strap and buckle to a lug on the

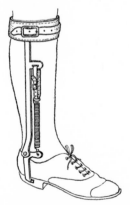

Fig. 61. Side steel and toe-raising spring

76

upper part of the side-iron. At its distal end the lower section has a spur, rectangular in cross-section, which fits a socket in the heel of the shoe. Thus the tension on the spring produces dorsiflexion of the foot (*see* Fig. 61).

This appliance is more acceptable than the toe-raising spring, but still produces wear on trousers and is somewhat bulky.

A more elegant derivative of this pattern is produced by Remploy, where the spring, which is much shorter and enclosed, is mounted on the posterior aspect of the side-iron immediately above the ankle hinge and is constantly under compression. Adjustment of tension is carried out readily by means of an Allen key turning a screw device on the upper end of the spring enclosure (*see* Fig. 62).

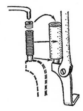

Fig. 62. Remploy type toe-raising appliance

(*c*) *Exeter type*

In common with other Exeter splints, the appliance is made of spring steel, circular in cross-section, forming the double side-irons and bearing a calf band proximally. At the level of the ankle each side-iron is shaped into two circular turns and continued distally to end as flat spurs. The turns at the ankle joint level allow plantar flexion to occur from the rest position which is in some 10 to 15 degrees of dorsiflexion (*see* Fig. 63).

In spite of these turns, some whipping of the side bars does occur during walking.

If this appliance fails, the fatigue fracture usually develops where the side-irons are bent at the beginning of the circular turns.

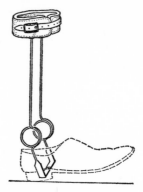

Fig. 63. Exeter type toe-raising spring

(*d*) *Stanmore type*

Double below-knee irons are used with a calf band proximally, and terminating distally with square spurs, each fitting a socket in the heel. The latter is spring loaded to produce dorsiflexion at rest, and the mechanism is totally enclosed.

The main difficulty in supply is the spring resistance which should be overcome easily by body weight, but experience in supplying the appliance enables the fitter to estimate the required strength of spring readily.

A less efficient type of the same basic design has round spurs and a helical spring set in the heel, but otherwise not

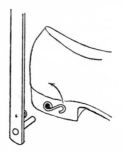

Fig. 64. Heel-spring pattern

78

enclosed. The end of the spring is formed into a hook which catches on the lower end of one of the side-irons. Here the difficulty of estimation of the spring strength is greater because of friction between the heel and the turns of the spring, and this is magnified by contamination with water and grit from the roads. In time it becomes very noisy in spite of repeated lubrication (*see* Fig. 64).

(*e*) *Posterior steel and insole*

A calf band supports a flat spring steel lying on the posterior aspect of the calf and terminating in an insole. Behind the ankle the spring deviates from the line of the leg, returning to it just below the ankle to lie against the heel and fit into the shoe. There is an angle of approximately 120° at this point, and it is here that fatigue fractures tend to occur (*see* Fig. 65).

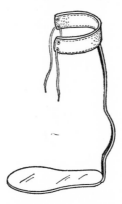

Fig. 65. Posterior spring and insole

EQUINUS FOOT

This may be an active equinus, the result of a spastic condition from any cause, or a passive equinus due to tight posterior structures. The foot is, therefore, held in the deformed position, either by muscle action or by contractures and hence it will be

79

impossible to achieve a plantigrade position until these forces have been overcome.

APPLIANCES

Night splints. These are obviously of prime importance. They are best made from one of the more recently developed plastics as this combines cheapness with cleanliness. It consists of a simple posterior gutter splint, with the angle between the calf and foot sections less than the corresponding angle on the

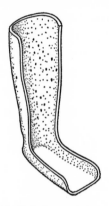

Fig. 66. Polythene night splint

patient. The appliance should be used every night, being bandaged firmly in position in an attempt to overcome the deformity and should be re-made as soon as the heel can be fully accommodated within that appliance. When full correction has been achieved by the appliance, it may be discontinued, but should be recommenced as soon as any degree of equinus develops (*see* Fig. 66).

Toe-raising spring. As described for foot-drop. In addition to suffering from the disadvantages previously mentioned, the force applied in an active equinus is too great for this type of appliance. One finds that the calf band is frequently pulled down the leg unless it is done up extremely tightly and this, in itself, could lead to discomfort. In addition, it may result in deformity of the shoe, producing hyperextension of the meta-tarsophalangeal joint. In view of these disadvantages, this type of appliance is best avoided.

Single or double side-irons

  (i) With back-stop as previously described. This suffers from the same disadvantage as when used for foot-drop, and indeed, one is even more likely to meet a patient whose quadriceps are weak and, therefore, 'knee-shooting' is more frequently seen.

 (ii) Flat spur with ankle hinge and side spring. It is likely that double springs will be necessary, but with this modification, this is probably the most satisfactory appliance.

(iii) Square spur incorporating coil spring (Stanmore pattern). Once the tension is correct, this is an extremely good appliance, but the initial adjustment can be difficult.

(iv) Posterior spring and insole. In view of the extreme forces applied in a spastic condition, this appliance has no place in the treatment of an active equinus foot.

In brief, the problems of fitting an appliance to a patient with foot-drop are even more marked when dealing with an active equinus foot. There is the constant problem of overcoming the forces of spastic calf muscles, especially if associated with weak quadriceps, which predispose the 'knee-shoot' and instability on hills and stairs.

GENU VALGUM

This condition is commonly seen at three ages:
(*a*) The young child who is frequently fat.
(*b*) Teenagers and
(*c*) The adult.

THE YOUNG CHILD

When sitting with knees extended and lower ends of thighs together, the distance between the medial malleoli exceeds 1 inch (2·5 cm.). At this age, the deformity is commonly associated with lax collateral ligaments of the knees, and, indeed, if the knees are pressed firmly together, it is common to find that the medial malleoli can, in fact, be approximated. When standing, however, the child usually has his feet a few inches apart, but his knees together and his body weight falling between his knees stretching the medial ligaments. The deformity is, therefore, more apparent than real.

Two methods of treatment are commonly used for this condition:

(i) *Wedges to inner border of soles and heels of shoes.* It is quite clear that the alteration in posture produced by this addition to the footwear is compensated by inversion of the foot at the subtaloid joint, and no corrective force can possibly be applied to the knees. This appliance, therefore, is of no value.

(ii) *Mermaid-type splints.* This appliance consists of two metal gutter splints, back-to-back which are inserted between the child's legs, straps being passed round the limb at the

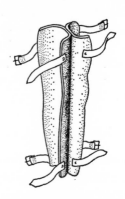

Fig. 67. Mermaid splints

level of the thigh and ankle. A moment's reflection will show that this simply stretches the lateral ligament of the knees and exacerbates the ligamentous laxity which is already present (*see* Fig. 67).

One must accept that there is no method of conservative treatment available for this type of deformity, but one should also accept that in the great majority of cases no treatment is necessary. If these children are watched at intervals of three to four months, one commonly sees that the distance between the medial malleoli when the knees are together does not increase, although if the angle between the thigh and the tibia remains the same, the distance should become greater because of increased length of leg. Reassurance to the parents is needed until the child reaches the age of 5 to 7 years and during this time, one usually finds that the deformity is corrected over a period of a very few months by growth.

THE TEENAGER

The second age at which the condition presents is usually in the early teens. The patient is frequently a short, fat female who has some 2 inches (5 cm.) to 3 inches (7·5 cm.) between her medial malleoli and no ligamentous laxity. One frequently finds that her mother has the same shape. The condition in itself, does not produce symptoms, but the patient or her mother is frequently worried about the appearance. One should then decide whether surgery is indicated to improve the appearance or to avoid later lateral compartment degeneration, but no appliance can be expected to correct the bone structure.

THE ADULT

The third age at which it presents is in patients over 30 years of age, when the patient, still overweight and with considerable genu valgum, begins to develop degenerative changes in the knees. This problem is clearly one of defective weight-bearing and will inevitably lead to osteoarthritis. It is best treated by corrective surgery.

TIBIAL TORSION

This abnormality, which is usually internal in direction, is commonly associated with one of the various forms of talipes. Denis Browne hobble splints and night boots, which are used for the latter condition, do attempt to correct the tibial torsion by eversion of the foot when in the splint, but the author has not seen any definite evidence of improvement which could not be explained by growth derotation. In theory, it would be possible to correct tibial torsion by applying an above-knee plaster, with the knee at 90 degrees and the foot plantigrade. This would undoubtedly apply a torsional strain on the tibia, but it is likely that the strain would be most effective in stretching the ligaments of the knee.

BOWED TIBIAE

It is common to see a baby of from three to twelve months old whose mother is worried because his legs are bowed. Careful examination usually shows that the tibia is quite straight and that the bowing is due to the distribution of muscle bulk and fat in a small leg. Carefully positioned anteroposterior X-rays will confirm this and reassurance is all that is required. Should a genuine case of bowed tibiae be found in the clinic, a Mermaid-type of night splint has been used, but with little success. It is usually wiser to resort to early manual osteoclasis.

GENU VARUM

It is uncommon to find genu varum which is not the result of bone disease or trauma. Corrective splints of the Mermaid type have been used and the result is that the medial ligament of the knee becomes lax. The only method of treatment likely to be of any value is surgical.

FIVE

Abnormalities of the Feet

TALIPES SPLINTS

Denis Browne and many others have devised appliances of several designs to correct the deformities which may be present in this group of congenital abnormalities. It is safe to say that the most persistent and potentially disabling deformities are found in talipes equino-varus, and the majority of the splints available are for use in this condition.

HOBBLE SPLINT

As described by Denis Browne the basic splint for each foot is shaped to the plan of five equal squares as shown in the diagram. The two squares to form the side-lever are bent to a right angle at the junction with the other three, and then curved to avoid pressure on the lateral malleolus, in to meet

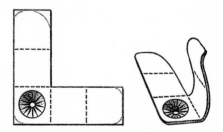

Fig. 68. Denis Browne hobble splint

the lower third of the leg, and the extreme tip curved out again to prevent the edge cutting in. The third square is drilled and dished to take a bolt which enables fixation to a correspondingly dished crossbar.

This device, if applied as intended, is capable of exerting corrective forces:

(*a*) valgus by felt packing,

(*b*) dorsiflexion by the side arm,

(*c*) external rotation by the crossbar.

Precise instructions for application are given in the original article and have been reiterated several times since then. The first essential is that each component of the composite deformity should be corrected by manipulation beginning distally and working proximally. Felt padding is then stuck to the plantar surface of the child's foot in a wedge thicker on the lateral aspect. The foot-piece is strapped to the foot, and at this stage it will be seen that the side-lever stands away from the leg and usually in a more anterior plane. When the side-lever is strapped to the leg, the foot will become everted and the equinus position corrected. Application of the crossbar is the final stage, external rotation being used to correct any medial torsion of the tibia.

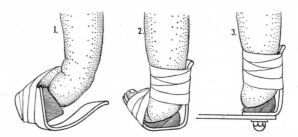

Fig. 69. Application of hobble splint

Each component of the basic splint has been modified in some way since the original description. Denis Browne has listed twelve of these alterations and produced valid criticisms of most of them. It is therefore recommended that the original design be used.

DENIS BROWNE NIGHT BOOTS

Based on the hobble-splint principle, the device consists of leather open-toed bootees fixed to a crossbar so that any degree of rotation may be selected. The bootee has a straight medial border to correct the adduction of the forefoot and often a strap passing across the front of the ankle, through slots in the heel to buckle posteriorly, so ensuring that the child's heel is held well down in the appliance.

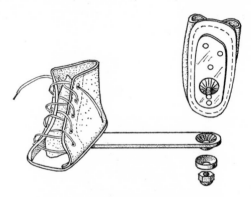

Fig. 70. Denis Browne night boots

Correction of the varus is a problem with this appliance. In the hobble splint it is achieved by sticking a felt wedge on to the child's foot and Denis Browne believed that this was necessary to avoid frictional changes on the skin. Clearly such a wedge cannot be reapplied every night and would be in the way if left in situ. The choice is then either to apply a felt wedge in the bootee, or to bend the crossbar to produce the valgus (*see* Fig. 70).

CALCANEUS NIGHT BOOT

Although described by Denis Browne for use in paralytic or spastic states the device may be useful in talipes conditions.

It consists of an open-toed leather bootee with a metal strip projecting from the posterior border of the heel. A posterior steel and calf band are attached to the metal strip through two simple hinges set at right angles to each other to allow dorsiflexion at the ankle and inversion or eversion at the subtaloid joint. At the upper limit of the bootee a leather strap encircles the leg and is attached to the posterior steel. Corrective forces are applied by a strap arising from the calf band passing through a loop on the radius bar and back to the calf band. The radius bar is a strip of metal pivoted on the sole of the bootee and capable of being fixed in varus or valgus. Thus tension on the strap from the calf band will pull the foot into inversion or eversion and also into calcaneus.

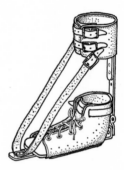

Fig. 71. Calcaneus night boot

In bilateral talipes equino-varus two of these appliances may be fixed together by a crossbar hinged to allow eversion, but which will hold the feet in external rotation.

HALLUX VALGUS

PATHOLOGY

On inspection, one can see valgus deviation of the big toe, commonly associated with rotation so that the plantar aspect of the big toe is applied to the second toe. Associated with the valgus deviation is stretching of the medial capsule and shortening of the lateral capsule. The sesamoids are displaced laterally and the extensor tendon can be seen to bow-string across the angle between the first metatarsal and the hallux.

ASSOCIATED DEFORMITIES

The deviation of the big toe leaves the head of the first metatarsal exposed and due to increased pressure from footwear an exostosis is formed on the medial aspect of the metatarsal head. Overlying this is a bursa which frequently becomes inflamed. The first metatarsal is frequently deviated away from the second, producing a metatarsus primus varus. The displacement of the big toe produces a secondary deformity of the second toe and may lie on the dorsal aspect of this digit which has a hammer deformity, or it may lie on the plantar aspect. In either event, the proximal interphalangeal joint of the second toe is prominent, and pressure from the shoe produces a corn at this site. One frequently sees pes planus anterior or a planovalgus deformity associated with hallux valgus. Thus this very common combination of conditions, seen particularly in aged ladies, is metatarsus primus varus and hallux valgus, with a bunion, hammer deformity of the second toe, pes planus anterior and a planovalgus foot.

AETIOLOGY

(a) *Familial.* It is very common to find a history of a similar deformity of the foot in other members of the family and this association is more common in females. Many papers have been written on the incidence of this condition and several authors have stressed that the metatarsus primus varus is the primary condition whereas other writers consider hallux valgus to occur first.

(b) *An acquired variety*, undoubtedly, is seen and this is probably related to the deformity of the foot produced by wearing tight and unsuitably shaped shoes or tight stockings.

TREATMENT

(a) *Strapping.* A strip of 1 inch (2·5 cm.) zinc-oxide strapping is applied to the foot in the following manner. It begins on the lateral aspect of the big toe, running round the tip of the terminal segment and along the medial border of the big toe. At this point, tension is applied to the strapping to correct the valgus position of the hallux. The strapping then continues along the medial border of the foot and round the heel. It is supported by circumferential strapping at the level of the proximal phalanx of the big toe and also at the level of the tarsometatarsal joint. This will maintain a mobile deformity in the correct position and has the advantage that it can be worn under the stockings, but the disadvantage that it needs frequent re-application (*see* Fig. 72).

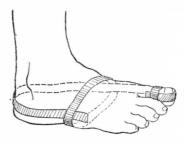

Fig. 72. Zinc oxide strapping for hallux valgus

(*b*) *Tubegauz.* A spica of Tubegauz applied over the big toe with a tail extending round the medial border of the foot will provide a correcting force, but tension must be applied to the medial tail of the bandage and this is maintained by circumferential strapping at the level of the tarsometatarsal joint. Owing to stretching of the Tubegauz, however, and the difficulty of maintaining traction, this method is not recommended.

(*c*) *Interdigital pegs.* Sponge rubber pegs are produced by several firms. These are meant to be inserted between the first and second toes. If the peg is not fixed to a sole-plate it is difficult to see how it can do anything more than increase the pressure on the second toe. If it is fixed to an insole, it can certainly correct the deformity, but it is not possible to wear this appliance with stockings or socks in position.

(*d*) *Elastic straps.* An elastic band some 3 inches (7·5 cm.) in width has been devised which is worn round the forefoot. A short cylinder of elastic to encircle the big toe is attached to the distal edge of the band, thus enclosing the big toe and forefoot in a spica-like support. The tension along the medial border of the elastic spica is expected to overcome the deforming force of extensor hallucis longus and flexor hallucis longus and it is difficult to imagine reasonably thin elastic having sufficient resilience to overcome these two powerful muscles working in unison.

(*e*) *Stanmore night splint.* This splint consists of a spring-steel lever extending from the medial aspect of the tip of the great toe along the medial border of the foot, round the heel and

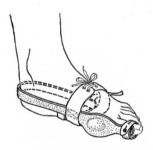

Fig. 73. Stanmore pattern of hallux valgus splint

along the lateral border of the foot to the level of the tarso-metatarsal joint. Circumferential straps are applied (*a*) round the big toe, (*b*) round the foot at the level of the tarsometatarsal joint. This appliance clearly can only be worn when the patient is unshod, and, therefore, its use is confined to night splints. It is difficult to see how its use would do more than stretch the contracted soft tissues and while it is useful as a post-operative appliance, it is unlikely to avoid the need for operation (*see* Fig. 73).

A variant of the splint made from sheet aluminium has been described by Lamber Moodie and this has a flange projecting from the plantar aspect of the appliance at the big-toe level extending into the first interdigital cleft.

H. H. Jordan, in *Orthopaedic Appliances: The Principles and Practice of Brace Construction* (1963), summarizes the position: 'We must realize it is not possible to correct a hallux valgus deformity of the foot by means of an orthopaedic appliance.'

HALLUX RIGIDUS

DESCRIPTION

This condition is an osteoarthritis of the first metatarso-phalangeal joint. The patient, therefore, complains of pain, stiffness, and swelling. The stiffness is usually worse after sitting still for any length of time but may wear off after walking about for a short period. As with any other form of degenerative arthritis, there is restriction of movement, but in hallux rigidus the first movement to be lost is that of dorsiflexion.

In walking normally, the big toe is passively dorsiflexed at the metatarsophalangeal joint, the angle of dorsiflexion varying with the length of stride and the height of heels being worn. Once the range of free dorsiflexion has decreased to an angle which is less than that passively produced during walking, the patient will experience pain in this part at each step. For a time he will compensate for the loss of movement by taking shorter steps, by wearing lower heels, or perhaps by walking with the hips externally rotated, the foot then rolling onto the inner border to avoid the painful movement. Eventually, however, these compensating methods fail and the patient may present complaining of pain either in the first metatarsophalangeal joint or in the dorsum of the foot.

DEFORMITY

On inspection, the first metatarsophalangeal joint is usually swollen and there may be an exostosis arising from the dorsal aspect of the first metatarsal head. This contrasts with the exostosis seen in hallux valgus where it arises from the medial aspect of the first metatarsal head. In hallux rigidus the exostosis is usually much smaller than in hallux valgus and, also, the base is relatively narrow, although it may still be capped by a bursa over which is hyperkeratotic skin. Occasionally, this bursa may become inflamed and may even suppurate and discharge to the surface, leaving a sinus. There is always some degree of restriction of movement of the first metatarsophalangeal joint, as described above.

At the time most patients present, plantar flexion is still present for a reasonable proportion of the normal range but dorsiflexion is usually completely absent. Compensating for this, there is frequently an increased range of dorsiflexion of the interphalangeal joint of the big toe.

CONSERVATIVE TREATMENT

The treatment of hallux rigidus must aim at either regaining the lost dorsiflexion or allowing the patient to walk without the need for dorsiflexion of the first metatarsophalangeal joint. There is no appliance available which will assist in the former method and one must, therefore, rely on techniques which avoid the painful movement.

(a) *Steel sole plate.* The insertion of a small steel plate between the layers of the sole and heel of the shoe will effectively prevent dorsiflexion of the metatarsophalangeal joints during heel and toe walking.

In a normal patient the foot acts as a lever, the fulcrum of which is at the head of the first metatarsal, the weight being applied at the talus and the force moving the lever being provided by the calf muscles at their insertion to the os calcis. If the first metatarsophalangeal joint becomes stiffened, the length of the lever is increased so that the fulcrum lies either at the head of the proximal phalanx if there is compensatory hyperextension of this joint, or at the pulp of the big toe. Since the force required to move a lever varies with the length of the lever, even a small increase in the length of the lever arm produces the need for application of a much greater force to move the lever and, therefore, the effort of walking with a steel sole plate is much greater than in the normal foot. The patient tends to avoid this extra effort by externally rotating the hips and rolling from the lateral border of the foot across the metatarsal heads, so producing a gait which has been described as 'ten to 2'. In time this gait will produce a planovalgus deformity of the foot.

(b) *Rocker sole.* The design of clogs is such that, with the curved sole, the wearer can roll forward on the clogs without the need for dorsiflexion at the metatarsophalangeal joints. A similar effect can be produced on shoes by the addition of several layers of leather between the two layers of the sole,

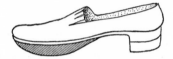

Fig. 74. Rocker sole

thus giving the plantar aspect of the sole a pronounced curve. With a shoe of this type the patient's body-weight rolls from the heel to the tip of the shoe and, in addition, the sole acts as a splint preventing flexion across its midpoint. The disadvantage is that the sole is usually at least $\frac{1}{2}$ inch (1·25 cm.) thick at the level of the metatarsophalangeal joints and, therefore, the heel of the shoe must be raised by an equivalent amount. Also, in unilateral hallux rigidus, a similar alteration must be made to the other shoe so that the patient can stand on an even base. This alteration of the shoe is heavy and is only applicable to the more sturdy variety of shoes, but does enable the wearer to walk heel and toe without increased effort (*see* Fig. 74.).

(c) *Metatarsal bars.* Two varieties of metatarsal bars are prescribed, outside and concealed.

An outside metatarsal bar consists of an extra layer of leather applied across the sole of the shoe on its plantar surface immediately behind the metatarsal heads which, if applied correctly, will be curved across the shoe to follow the skeletal shape. When newly applied, a metatarsal bar will produce a rocker-like effect but it rapidly wears down to lie flush with the sole of the shoe anterior to the metatarsal

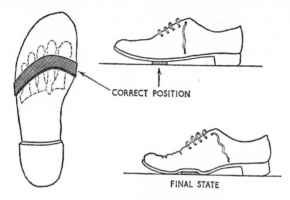

Fig. 75. Metatarsal bar

heads and is, therefore, ineffective. In addition, if the shoe is not sturdy enough to take the localized strain imposed upon it, the sole becomes deformed so that its inner surface is lifted up, producing the effect of a metatarsal insole, the metatarsal heads being supported from inside the shoe but there is no rocker effect on the outside. Indeed, this is probably the way in which metatarsal bars (*see* Fig. 75) are of value in other conditions of the foot (see pes planus anterior).

Concealed metatarsal bars have the same design but are placed between the two layers of the sole. They, therefore, do not wear down as readily as do the outside bars but the resistance to deformity of the sole is reduced because only one layer of leather is between the bar and the foot and, therefore, the likelihood of shoe deformity is greater. In effect, a metatarsal bar does produce a minor degree of rocker sole until deformity of the shoe occurs but even before the deformity is present, the bar is usually inadequate and ineffective.

CONCLUSION

It will be seen that of the above appliances the one most likely to be of value is the rocker sole, although its application is limited to those patients who are willing to wear a heavy shoe with a thick sole. The appliance looks incongruous on light footwear but equally this type of footwear cannot be used for metatarsal bars or steel sole plates. Surgical methods of treatment are more satisfactory for hallux rigidus but the above appliances may be of help when operation is contra-indicated.

SHORT FIRST METATARSAL[1]

This condition, extensively investigated by Drs. Harris and Beath in members of the Canadian Forces, has been implicated in many conditions which produce symptoms in the forefoot. It has been blamed for pes planus anterior, planovalgus feet and Morton's metatarsalgia, which is a condition in which the heads of the 2nd, 3rd and 4th metatarsals produce pressure on the digital nerves, and, therefore, pain radiating to adjacent sides of two toes. In their paper, however, they have demonstrated very ably that the incidence of these symptoms is not greater in a patient with a short first metatarsal than in any other patient. Nevertheless, the clinician may feel that some form of correction is indicated in a given case and the following appliances can be expected to prove satisfactory:

(1) Rose's insole.
(2) Metatarsal pad.
(3) Metatarsal insole. (For details of all of these, *see* pes planus anterior, page 106.)

[1] 'The Short First Metatarsal' Harris and Beath (1949) *J. B. J. S.*, 31A, 553.

HYPERMOBILE FIRST METATARSAL

It is relatively common, particularly in young patients, and certainly with those with Ehlers-Danlos syndrome. In the normal foot there is a small range of passive dorsiflexion and plantar flexion of the first metatarsal occurring at the medial cuneiform-metatarsal joint. In this condition, the range of movement exceeds that normally found and, in extreme cases, may reach 30 degrees. When weight-bearing, therefore, the first metatarsal is passively dorsiflexed and to secure stability the foot moves into eversion, thus producing one of the varieties of planovalgus foot. It is possible by a muscular effort on the part of the patient to correct eversion of the foot, but this correction is not maintained on normal walking. It is necessary, therefore, to provide a passive supporting insole in order to avoid the formation of a fixed planovalgus foot. The appliances likely to be of value are the various forms of valgus insoles which are all described in the section on planovalgus feet, or Rose's insole which is described in the section on pes planus anterior (page 107).

METATARSUS PRIMUS VARUS

DESCRIPTION

In the normal foot it is obvious that the breadth at the base of the metatarsals is less than at their heads. The metatarsal axes, therefore, diverge from one another. The angle between the axes of the first and second metatarsals has been the subject of many papers over the past twenty years and the upper limit of normal has not been established to the satisfaction of many anatomists. However, most writers would agree that divergence in excess of 10 degrees is abnormal.

Lapidus has written several papers dealing with this deformity and he is of the opinion that a deviation in excess of 10 degrees is normal during foetal development and its persistence into adult life is simply a failure of the normal progression. He

97

compares the human foot with that of apes and monkeys, finding that arboreal creatures have a wider angle between the first and second metatarsals than have terrestrial animals.

Other workers consider that metatarsus primus varus is an acquired condition, developing during childhood.

From the clinician's point of view, it certainly seems to be more common in the 14-year-old girl than in a child of 10 years younger. Some orthopaedic surgeons consider that it is the cause of hallux valgus but others maintain that hallux valgus leads to a varus position of the first metatarsal. The clinical impression gained in school clinics suggests that either can exist without the other and that neither is an essential precursor of the other.

CONSERVATIVE TREATMENT

The problem is to prevent an increase in the distance between the first and second metatarsal heads. The obvious way of doing this is by wearing a firm strap round the foot at the level of the metatarsal necks, and this is provided easily by a metatarsal pad. Since this loses its elasticity after a few weeks, however, it is unlikely to be of any lasting value unless renewed at frequent intervals.

PHYSIOTHERAPY

The only muscle likely to exert any restraining effect on the first metatarsal is adductor hallucis and it is difficult to see how selective exercise of this small muscle deep in the sole of the foot could be achieved.

PLANOVALGUS FEET

This deformity is the so-called 'flat-foot'. The term, although used so commonly, is strictly not correct in that the arch of the foot is frequently preserved, but on superficial examination, the appearance suggests that the arch is flattened. Careful inspection, however, shows that the deformity is eversion of the foot at the talonavicular and talocalcaneal joints and when viewed from the posterior aspect, the heel is seen to be in valgus, the medial border of the foot approaching the ground in the same way that a bucket handle approaches the side of a bucket when released from the hand. Excessive weight is taken along the medial border of the foot and when footprints in the weight-bearing position are taken, the normal concavity along the medial border of the foot is no longer present. The skin may be in contact with the ground, but the bony arch of the foot can still be present in its normal form.

If the shoe habitually worn by a patient with planovalgus deformity is examined, it will be seen that the weight is taken along the medial border of the sole and the top line of the shoe deviates towards the medial side. In other words, when viewed from above, the axis of the opening of the shoe is not in line with the shoe, but deviated medially. If this deflection is carried to an extreme, the structure of the shoe is broken down over the mid-point of the longitudinal arch (*see* Fig. 95, p. 131).

COMPLICATIONS

Shortening of the soft tissues on the lateral side of the foot and ankle occurs so that it may not be possible to correct the valgus position of the heel while maintaining full dorsiflexion of the foot. Faulty alignment in the tarsus will lead to degeneration in associated joints.

ASSOCIATED CONDITIONS

Hallux valgus, metatarsus primus varus and pes planus anterior are all commonly seen.

AETIOLOGY

This condition is very commonly seen in small children aged between 2 and 5 years and they frequently have lax ligaments in their knee joints, giving apparent genu valgum. This is so common as to be almost physiological in this age-group. If children are watched, without any form of treatment, but are encouraged to run about normally, the condition usually corrects spontaneously by the age of 5 years. It is probable, therefore, that this is simply a phase of development in which their body-weight exceeds their muscle-power and with the loss of puppy-fat and with the increase of activity at the time of starting school, the deformity is overcome naturally.

The next age-group in which this is commonly seen is in the 10 to 15 years group, whose parents complain that they wear shoes out rapidly and are often disheartened at not being able to run as fast as their fellows at school. At this age, the foot is still mobile and fixed contractions have not yet developed. The heel can be placed in the normal position under the talus and with concentration, they are usually able actively to maintain the arch for a short period.

The third group is in adult life when the deformity may still be mobile, but is frequently fixed and sometimes symptomless.

APPLIANCES

In the young child nothing needs to be done since normal activities in the great majority of cases result in spontaneous correction. If it is decided that treatment is needed, several methods are available.

Wedge heel. A wedge inserted on the medial side of the heel, with or without a wedge on the medial side of the sole, may correct the deformity until body-weight damages the strengthening inserts in the shoe construction. If wedging is to be carried out in the heels, this is best applied to leather heels several layers from that surface in contact with the ground as this facilitates repair of the shoes in the future (*see* Fig. 76). However, with the increased use of plastics and synthetic rubbers in the construction of children's shoes, this possibility is rapidly receding and one has to rely on a wedge of rubber stuck on the surface. In most children, this wears off within two or three weeks and must be frequently replaced. Cork wedges may be inserted inside the shoe at the heel, but these are impossible to keep in place unless they are stuck in position.

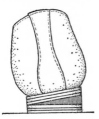

Fig. 76. Wedged heel

Insoles. Many types of insoles have been devised, both full length and three-quarter. They may be subdivided into two groups, active and passive.

The best example of the active insole was described by Whitman and consists of a metal arch support bearing flanges on its medial and lateral borders, the lateral flange extending up the side of the os calcis in such a way that the heel is gripped between the medial and the lateral flanges. Its shape is such that the os calcis is held in the normal position (*see* Fig. 77).

Fig. 77. Whitman's insole

The patient is instructed that when walking, he should throw his weight on to the outer side of his feet. This presses on the outer flange thus lifting the medial side of the sole plate against the foot. If, when walking in this way, the patient turns his toes outwards, he produces pain, and, therefore, tends to adopt the heel-toe gait. The function of this appliance is reminiscent of the kugeleinlage described by Spitz which consists of a leather insole on which is mounted a marble underneath the medial arch of the foot. So long as the patient with this appliance maintains the arch actively, there is no discomfort, but when he allows the arch to fall, the marble presses on the underneath of the foot and he instinctively draws it away. This is probably the most effective way of maintaining an arch although by far the most uncomfortable.

Passive supports of the foot are simply props which hold the foot in the desired position without any effort on the part of the patient. They are usually made from, or covered in, leather and there are pads along the medial margin extending two-thirds of the way across the foot. Some have a flange which

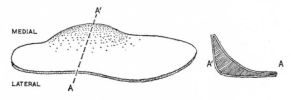

Fig. 78. Valgus insole

projects up the medial side of the foot and is expected to support the first metatarsal and cuneiform. Since this flange is usually made of thin leather, its long-term effect is negligible. The applied pad on most of these insoles consists of rubber or felt, covered with leather (*see* Fig. 78).

The important fact to consider when advising an appliance of this nature is the best shape of the arch which can be achieved without discomfort. If a patient has a rigid flat foot, any attempt at reforming an arch will inevitably produce pain. It is wise, therefore, to ensure that any prop provided does not over-correct the deformity.

One must also ensure that the structure of that prop is such that it will not pack down after a few weeks. Thus, the best combination that has been found to support a heavy man is a shaped metal insole provided on its undersurface with a pad of solid rubber. In theory, this should be an excellent appliance, but in practice it is not possible to have these metal insoles shaped accurately to a given foot. A compromise can often be

achieved by making the insole of a firm plastic to a cast of the
foot and sticking sheet rubber in layers on the undersurface,
trimming it to produce a contour which approximates to the
shape of the inner surface of the shoe.

A shaped heel-socket made of fibre-glass has been devised by
Helfet with the aim of gripping the heel and correcting its
position by a plantar wedge which is integral with the heel
grip. This appliance is worn inside the shoe, but by its nature
is so thick that a larger size of shoe is essential (*see* Fig. 79).

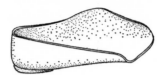

Fig. 79. Helfet's insole

Experience with this appliance shows that it does correct the
deformity very well provided that the original cast on which
the fibre-glass is shaped is an accurate representation of the
foot. During use, there is inevitably some movement of the heel
within the socket and this small range of movement is sufficient
to produce frictional changes in the skin. The movement of the
os calcis on the fatty plantar tissues of the heel is sufficient to
allow a small degree of eversion to occur and this movement
thousands of times a day does produce rubbing at the anterior
margin of the appliance. Indeed, it is not uncommon for bursae
to develop over the medial border of the navicular and although
these usually subside rapidly when the appliance is no longer
worn, it is possible that the effect is as much due to Spitz's
kugeleinlage as to the mechanical corrective position of the
appliance.

Floated heel. This consists of prolongation of the heel in a
medial direction and tends to correct the valgus position of the
heel provided the heel of the shoe grips the os calcis firmly.
(*See* Adaptations of Footwear, p. 135.)

An elongated (Thomas) heel is often used and is copied in a minor
way by at least one shoe manufacturer. This is a prolongation

of the heel along the medial border of the shoe to the level of the waist. Its effect is best seen when the eversion of the foot is so great that the deviation of body-weight to the medial side of the shoe is sufficient to destroy the normal arch of the shoe (*see* **Fig.** 80).

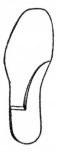

Fig. 80. Thomas elongated heel

The destruction of the shoe is effectively prevented by the Thomas heel but because of the movement which occurs between even a well-fitting shoe and the foot, it is difficult to see how any correcting force can be transmitted to the foot. This is also true of the use of wedges in shoes except when they are new and the heel counter is firm and closely fitting. In general, I think it is fair to say that these appliances can all act as suitable props to hold the foot in a corrected position, but one must expect them to have little curative value. It may well be that, in the adult, simple propping up is all that is required and under these circumstances, these appliances fulfil their function.

PES PLANUS ANTERIOR

SYMPTOMS

The patient will probably complain of pain on the forefoot or on the plantar surface of the forefoot, perhaps radiating down the adjacent borders of two toes. He may also complain of thickening of the skin on the plantar surface of the foot and there is frequently generalized aching over the dorsum of the foot. It is thought that this is the result of muscle strain because of an altered walking pattern.

APPEARANCE

In the normal foot at rest, the pillars of the anterior transverse arch are formed by the heads of the first and fifth metatarsal heads, the intermediate metatarsal heads lying at a slightly higher level. During weight-bearing, however, these metatarsal heads descend to lie on the same horizontal plane as the pillars of the arch, but investigation of the load taken by the metatarsal heads when standing has shown that the second, third and fourth metatarsals bear a smaller proportion of the body-weight than do the first and fifth. Pes planus anterior is an alteration of this normal distribution of weight in which the second, third and fourth metatarsals take a higher proportion of weight than is usual, and indeed, may even take the majority of the body-weight. Work hypertrophy of the skin under the affected metatarsals produces the common callosities which may form either an oval area under a single metatarsal head or a reniform area underlying three metatarsal heads. If the patient complains of 'shooting' pains radiating along adjacent borders of the toes, pressing between metatarsal heads will frequently reproduce this symptom which is the result of pressure on a digital nerve as it lies between metatarsal heads. If one is in doubt about this involvement of the digital nerve, an anaesthetic block to the nerve at the level of the metatarsal shafts will always relieve the 'shooting' pain, but the discomfort of increased weight-bearing under the metatarsal heads will remain.

ASSOCIATED DEFORMITIES

It is common to see clawed toes, perhaps with dorsal dislocation of metatarsophalangeal joints. Hallux valgus and metatarsus primus varus are frequently present and pes cavus from any cause is always associated with pes planus anterior.

COMPLICATIONS

The only complication of note is Morton's metatarsalgia, i.e. pressure on a digital nerve as it passes between the metatarsal heads. It is this which leads to the pain radiating down the adjacent borders of two toes.

PATHOLOGY

(a) Muscle in balance from any cause.
(b) A period of prolonged bed-rest with insufficient rehabilitation, especially if there is an injury to a lower limb. In this event, however, it is likely that the side affected will be that of the fracture, or if bilateral, the changes will be more marked on the previously injured side.

APPLIANCES

All the appliances available are intended to relieve the additional weight-bearing of the middle three metatarsal heads by increased pressure under the shafts of those metatarsals.
Metatarsal pads. Two varieties of these exist. The first, and most satisfactory, can be added to the shoe and consists of a pad of felt perhaps covered with leather stuck to the inner aspect of the sole. This should be placed in such a way that it lies immediately behind the metatarsal heads and of such a height that it reduces the weight borne by those structures. The pads of course, must be inserted in each pair of shoes that the patient has.

Removable metatarsal pads consist of a small pad of felt or sponge rubber covered with leather attached to which is an elastic strap which passes round the forefoot. When worn it is unable to move towards the toes because of the presence of the metatarsal heads and its lateral displacement is restricted by the first and fifth metatarsal heads on either side.

Its posterior displacement, however, is limited solely by the tension in the elastic straps and it is unlikely that this, even when new, has sufficient tension to prevent displacement when walking. If the appliance is worn under the sock, it is more stable than when worn over the sock, but in either position it is unlikely to remain in place for long.

Fig. 81. Metatarsal pad

Metatarsal insoles. These structures consist of an insole of three-quarter or full length (*see* Figs. 82 and 83) in which is built the felt or sponge rubber pad. Movement of the insole within the shoe is prevented by the insole itself abutting against the upper and it must of course be made so that the pad lies immediately behind the metatarsal heads and lifts them sufficiently to

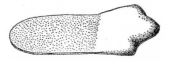

Fig. 82. Three-quarter metatarsal insole

relieve weight. They may be made of plastic or metal and provided that the pad is sufficiently incompressible, either of these is satisfactory. It must be stressed, however, that a heavy person will compress a pad far more than one would expect and the writer has seen metal insoles broken under the weight of a man weighing 15 stones.

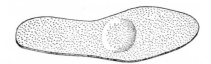

Fig. 83. Full-length metatarsal insole

Rose's insole. This type of insole may be three-quarter or full length, but the pad is of such a size that it completely fills in the transverse and longitudinal arches of the foot. Thus the pad extends from the metatarsal necks to the anterior margin of the os calcis and lies under all the metatarsals, but is manufactured in such a way that its maximum height in the longitudinal plane is about ½ inch (1·25 cm.) behind the metatarsal necks and its maximal height in the transverse plane is under the second metatarsal shaft (*see* Fig. 84).

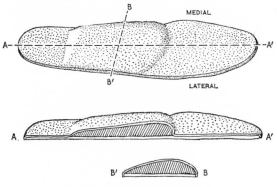

Fig. 84. Rose's insole

Metatarsal bars. There are two varieties of metatarsal bars available: the surface ones and those which are concealed. The surface type is a curve of several layers of leather applied to the sole of the shoe just behind the metatarsal head level. The concealed variety is a similar-shaped structure applied between the layers of the sole (*see* Fig. 85).

When one is ordering an appliance of this nature, one must consider very carefully the needs of the patient. If one accepts that relief of symptoms can be achieved by reduction of weight-bearing by the intermediate metatarsal heads, one must consider how this can be achieved by the use of a metatarsal bar.

If one imagines a patient who has a shoe, the sole of which is so stiff that his body-weight does not deform the sole when a metatarsal bar is in situ, it is difficult to see how the bar can relieve weight from the metatarsal heads. If one accepts that no weight is taken from the metatarsal heads under these conditions, one would obviously not order metatarsal bars.

If you consider, then, a patient with a shoe, the sole of which is deformed by his body-weight when wearing metatarsal bars, one must think what happens to the bonding material between the two layers of the sole when they are deformed. In either case, the upper layer of the sole is forced into a sigmoid

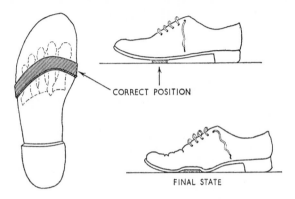

CORRECT POSITION

FINAL STATE

Fig. 85. Metatarsal bar

curve, the middle third of which is convex upwards and its course is, therefore, longer than that of the lower layer of the sole, but these two layers have been applied and bonded together with the upper surface concave. Therefore, there will be considerable strain on the bonding material and in the case of sewn soles, it is almost certain that the stitching will give way. It is difficult to see how an effective relief of symptoms can be achieved without irreparably damaging the structure of the shoes. Certainly, with the single layer of sole present in most ladies' shoes, one can only use a surface bar and the sole of the shoe is so thin that deformity of the shoe is inevitable. It means, therefore, that the patient either uses shoes which are not deformed by the bar, and, therefore, the bar is ineffective or the shoes must be destroyed by the bar if they are to produce relief of symptoms. Experience has shown that an equal relief of symptoms can be achieved by the use of metatarsal insoles and, therefore, it would seem that metatarsal bars for pes planus anterior are unnecessary.

BUNIONS

DESCRIPTION

A bunion is a bursa overlying an exostosis on the medial aspect of the first metatarsophalangeal joint. It is usually associated with hallux valgus, which in turn may be associated with a varus displacement of the first metatarsal. The bunion frequently becomes inflamed, leading to intermittent swelling, redness and increased pain, which may progress to discharge of purulent material. If, following infection, the skin and the lining of the bursa become continuous, there will be a persistent discharge of serous fluid, which will not heal until surgical intervention has taken place.

A bunionette is a similar condition which occurs on the lateral aspect of the fifth metatarsal head and is commonly associated with a valgus displacement of the fifth metatarsal and a varus deformity of the fifth toe.

CONSERVATIVE TREATMENT

Apart from methods available for correction of the associated deformities, the only method of treatment is avoidance of pressure and friction over the established bunion. This can be achieved by ring pads or suitably shaped sponge rubber pads which may be worn in shoes broader than are normally needed for that foot. It is usually simpler to arrange for shoes to be made to measure since these can be constructed of soft material with plenty of room for the sponge rubber pads to be accommodated.

The patient's normal shoes can be adapted by replacement of an eliptical section of the upper by a sheet of soft leather but this is a makeshift method which will not stand up to hard wear. Sewing soft leather into a relatively rigid upper produces great strains on the inserted material, which frequently tears round the stitch holes. In addition, there are problems of waterproofing and in the long term it is probably better to provide shoes made to measure at the first instance.

It must be stressed that these methods of treatment are purely palliative and no method short of surgery can be expected to remove the bunion or its underlying exostosis.

HAMMER TOE

DESCRIPTION

A hammer toe deformity is one in which there is hyperextension of the metatarsophalangeal joint, hyperflexion of the proximal interphalangeal joint and hyperextension of the distal interphalangeal joint. This condition may arise because of muscular imbalance from any cause or from tightly fitting stockings or shoes. Commonly, however, no cause can be found. In the early stages, passive correction of the deformity is easy but the deformity eventually becomes fixed. It is usual for the lateral slips of the extensor expansion to become displaced to the plantar side of the axis of the proximal interphalangeal joint and, therefore, to work as flexors, so perpetuating the deformity.

ASSOCIATED DEFORMITIES

There is usually a corn over the dorsal aspect of the proximal interphalangeal joint which arises because of friction and pressure on the shoe. It is common to see a hammer toe deformity as a complication of hallux valgus and, in this case, the displaced big toe will be found to lie on the dorsal aspect of the distal interphalangeal joint of the deformed second toe. It may also occur as a complication of Freiberg's infraction.

CONSERVATIVE TREATMENT

The need is to straighten the deformed toe and to hold it straight if this is possible. Relief may also be gained by removal of pressure from the flexed proximal interphalangeal joint.

(a) *Strapping*. Correction of the deformity by application of zinc-oxide strapping by the method shown in the diagram, may be of value in the early stages but needs to be reapplied at frequent intervals for many months. It is possible that

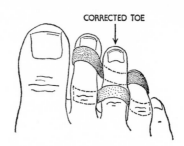

CORRECTED TOE

Fig. 86. Strapping for hammer toe

this method may delay the onset of a threatened deformity or even prevent it but application will need to be continued indefinitely. It is unlikely to be of any lasting value in an established deformity.

(b) *Ring pads*. Felt pads applied round the main pressure area will relieve the symptoms of the corn but will have no effect on the basic deformity (*see* Fig. 87).

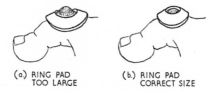

(a.) RING PAD TOO LARGE   (b.) RING PAD CORRECT SIZE

Fig. 87. Ring pad

(c) *Sponge rubber pads*, applied between or beneath the toes, have been described and frequently prescribed. Since they are worn on the plantar aspect of the toe, it is difficult to see how they can allow the toe to straighten. In straightening of the toe the proximal interphalangeal joint approaches the sole of the shoe and if this space is taken up by a sponge rubber pad, correction of the deformity manifestly becomes impossible.

(d) *Night splints*, consisting of a sole plate which is perforated at the level of the toes and which bears straps passing across the dorsum of the toes to be tightened after insertion of the foot, may have some value in the early case or post-operatively but it is doubtful whether they are of any value for the established deformity (*see* Fig. 88).

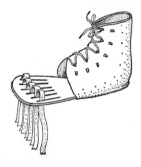

Fig. 88. Hammer toe night splint (Lambrinudi pattern)

CONCLUSION

Operation may be postponed by assiduous use of one of the above methods in the early case and may be avoided altogether if the patient is willing to wear shoes made to measure with plenty of toe space so that pressure over the proximal inter-phalangeal joint is avoided altogether. It is doubtful whether any of the methods listed above will cure the established condition.

CLAWED TOES

DESCRIPTION

The most commonly seen deformity involves the lateral four toes of each foot and consists of hyperextension of the metatarso-phalangeal joints and flexion of the interphalangeal joints. The hyperextension may be such that dislocation occurs. The deformity is frequently the result of muscle imbalance resulting from poliomyelitis, Friedreich's ataxia etc. and in these conditions it is common to have a similar deformity of the great toe. In most cases, however, no underlying cause can be found. Clawing of a single toe may be present and this is frequently seen as a complication of Freiberg's infraction, although as in the multiple cases, it is usually idiopathic.

ASSOCIATED DEFORMITIES

It is common to find either pes planus anterior or pes cavus present.

COMPLICATIONS

Corns frequently develop over the interphalangeal joints and also at the tips of the toes. At the latter site they are particularly troublesome since they lie adjacent to the free edge of the nail, and are subjected to direct pressure at each step. In the advanced cases there seems to be very little soft tissue between the terminal phalanx and the thickened skin of the corn and this area will be extremely tender.

CONSERVATIVE TREATMENT

(1) *Sling strapping* as described for hammer toe deformity is frequently demonstrated for home application. This will correct the deformity in many early cases but it is doubtful whether cure can be achieved by this means (*see* Fig. 86, p. 112).

(2) *Ring pads* for protection of corns will relieve the symptoms of the corns themselves but have no curative effect on the basic deformity (*see* Fig. 87, p. 112).

(3) *Sponge rubber pads* which are worn within the socks to fill up the space under the concavity of the toes will lift the tips of the toes clear of the shoe and, therefore, reduce the frequency of

terminal corns but it is difficult to see how they can have any curative effect on the clawing. Indeed, since they produce elevation of the head of the proximal phalanx of each toe, it is probable that they will exacerbate the hyperextension of the metatarsophalangeal joint and increase the tendency towards dislocation of these joints. They will also increase the pressure of the proximal interphalangeal joint on the upper of the shoe.

(4) *Metatarsal supports.* If a foot with clawed toes has pressure applied under the necks of the metatarsals, it can be seen that flexion of the metatarsophalangeal joints and extension of the interphalangeal joints occurs. The effect of this pressure is to mimic contraction of the intrinsic muscles of the foot. Additional support for the metatarsal necks, therefore, is an effective means of diminishing the clawing. This pressure under the metatarsal necks can be produced by a variety of appliances.

(a) *Metatarsal pads.* A metatarsal pad consists of an oval of felt, sponge rubber or some similar material, thicker at one end than the other and enclosed within an envelope of leather to which is fixed an elastic strap passing round the forefoot. When used, this pad is applied to the foot in such a way that the thicker end lies immediately behind the heads of the middle three metatarsals and the elastic strap passes round the forefoot just behind the head of the first metatarsal. The appliance is worn underneath the sock, which helps to prevent displacement of the pad as the foot is inserted into the shoe. During use, displacement forwards and to either side is prevented by the metatarsal heads and displacement towards the heel is prevented only by the tightness of the strap round the forefoot. In practice, this strap rapidly loses its elasticity and posterior shift of the appliance is common (*see* Fig. 81, p. 107).

(b) *Metatarsal insoles.* These work in the same way as do metatarsal pads but because of the stabilizing effect of the insole itself, migration within the shoe is less commonly seen. The insole, of course, is not worn under the sock (*see* Figs. 82 and 83, p. 107).

(c) *Metatarsal bars.* These have been described in the section dealing with hallux rigidus. They are probably effective because they produce secondary deformity of the sole of the shoe, which raises a ridge behind the metatarsal heads. Because of the destructive effect on the shoe, this method is, although effective, undesirable (*see* Fig. 85, p. 109).

OPINION

In the early case of clawed toes in which passive correction can be achieved, it may well be that the use of these appliances will prevent a fixed deformity developing. It is possible that with the use of suitable physiotherapy, the need for appliances may be avoided altogether, but in the established and fixed deformity, no conservative method is likely to be of any value.

CORNS

DESCRIPTION

A corn is an area of hyperkeratosis in the centre of which is a semi-translucent spot consisting of compressed keratin. The condition arises as a result of pressure and/or friction applied over two bony prominences separated by a narrow gap. Thus a corn is seen over a prominent joint which is subjected to pressure from tight footwear or stockings.

It is extremely common to see a patient, usually a young woman, who complains of painful feet, and on inspection there will be a valgus deformity of the big toe and varus deformities of the remaining toes. Over each of the interphalangeal joints one can commonly see a corn and inspection of the footwear will show deformity of the upper at a site which corresponds to each of these corns. It is also frequent to find the same patient wearing stockings which constrict the toes and which produce the deviation already mentioned. There is great difficulty in persuading most of these patients to wear larger shoes and stockings, although, in fairness, one must note that these patients frequently have feet which are on the large side of normal and since our society tends to equate small feet with beautiful feet, one must sympathize with these ladies who do not wish to wear shoes of their correct size. It is also difficult to find the larger size of shoe readily available in pleasing styles and many patients will complain that they are unable to find shoes which fit.

CONSERVATIVE TREATMENT

It can readily be seen that any method which removes pressure from a corn will reduce its symptoms and in time it will disappear without surgical interference.

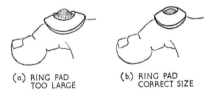

(a.) RING PAD   (b.) RING PAD
TOO LARGE   CORRECT SIZE

Fig. 89. Ring pad

The first necessity, therefore, is attention to footwear. Carefully chosen shoes must be bought, which not only leave room for the toes, but also room for the toes to move. The shoes must be fitted both with the patient seated and when standing and walking and this is preferably done at the end of the day since the feet will then be at their largest. Adequate room in the stockings is essential since enclosure within nylon stockings can produce as cramping an effect as tight leather shoes.

Local treatment for the corn is best provided by the use of ring pads but care must be taken to see that the pad is thick enough to avoid all pressure from footwear over the centre of the corn and that the hole in the centre is small enough to prevent the ring pad from sliding down the sides of the flexed interphalangeal joint, thus destroying the ring effect (*see* Fig. 89).

OVERRIDING FIFTH TOE

This is a congenital anomaly in which the fifth toe is elevated and deviated medially so that it lies on the dorsal aspect of the fourth toe. In addition, it is usually smaller than normal, flattened obliquely, and with a small hypoplastic nail. The obliquity of its shape is frequently said to be due to pressure of footwear, but, indeed, the full deformity can be seen in the new-born baby.

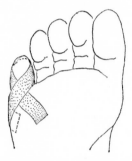

Fig. 90. Strapping for overriding fifth toe

Providing the subject is willing to wear shoes which have plenty of room for the toe in its abnormal position, the condition does not produce symptoms. However, many young mothers are distressed over the position of this toe and request that something should be done to correct the deformity. It must be clearly put to them at the beginning that this toe is hypoplastic and even if replaced in its normal position, will still not appear as a normal toe. It is theoretically possible that if the toe can be held in its correct position, the tight structures on the dorsi-medial aspect of the foot, i.e. skin, extensor tendon and capsule, will in due course adapt their length to fit the corrected position, but it must be frankly admitted that the author has never yet seen a parent who will persevere with the passive correction long enough to allow these changes to take place.

The solution, therefore, is to carry out one of the several operations which have been described for correction of this deformity, but in the post-operative phase, it is frequently helpful to maintain the position of the toe by the application of a strip of $\frac{1}{2}$ inch (1·25 cm.) zinc oxide strapping which is applied to the foot in the following manner. It begins on the plantar aspect of the foot under the head of the fourth metatarsal passing round the lateral border of the little toe, encircling it and finally being applied to the lateral aspect of the foot along the line of the fifth metatarsal. It will be seen, therefore, that this applies a force on the little toe tending to deviate it in a plantar and lateral direction, in fact, bisecting the angle made between the two overlapping strips of strapping (*see* Fig. 90).

INGROWING TOENAILS

DESCRIPTION

Two varieties of ingrowing toenails occur—(i) congenital; (ii) acquired.

(i) *Congenital.* In this variety the nail is usually small and its transverse curve in excess of normal. The patient is frequently stout, with fleshy feet, and the nail is set between fleshy folds of moist skin. Because of the increased transverse curve which, in an extreme case, may approximate to a semicircle, the free end of the nail at its margins presses into the soft tissue at the tip of the toe and this pressure is increased at each pace forward.

(ii) *Acquired.* In this variety of ingrowing toenail, the shape of the nail is normal. The main fault is that when cutting the toenails, the margins of the free end are cut back in a curve as is usual for fingernails, and during weight-bearing the soft tissues of the pulp are pressed up to lie above the level of the shortened nail. At each pace forward then, this soft tissue is pushed on to the free edge of the nail and this traumatic effect rapidly produces hyperaemia, oedema and, therefore, increased pressure. In time the skin becomes excoriated and infected, leading to further hyperaemia and oedema. Granulation tissue forms at the margins of the nail and there is a purulent discharge. The whole area becomes wet, soggy and swollen (*see* Fig. 91).

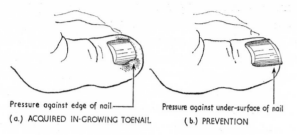

Pressure against edge of nail ————

(a.) ACQUIRED IN-GROWING TOENAIL

Pressure against under-surface of nail

(b.) PREVENTION

Fig. 91. Ingrowing toenail (acquired type)

CONSERVATIVE TREATMENT

Congenital. The main problem here is that the nail is surrounded by rather fat tissue. It may be possible to protect this soft tissue from the sharp free end of the nail until the nail has grown to project beyond the end of the pulp. When this has been done, weight-bearing simply presses the pulp tissues against the under-surface of the nail and no harm results. The use of pads of cottonwool inserted at frequent intervals under the free end of the nail may suffice. If these fail because of their bulk, it is

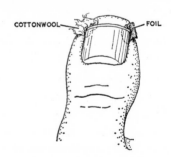

COTTONWOOL

FOIL

Fig. 92. Conservative management of ingrowing toenail

possible to make a small shield of aluminium foil, such as is used to cover the tops of milk bottles. A strip of this cut to fit under the free edge of the nail may provide sufficient protection to allow the nail to grow without excoriation (*see* Fig. 92).

Acquired. In this variety, the same techniques may be used with good effect. The main need here is to teach the patient the cause of the condition, to tell him that it is not really an ingrowing toenail but the soft tissues are being pushed onto the end of a normal nail. Most patients will readily accept this explanation, particularly if it is accompanied by diagrams, and can see the need to allow the nail to grow. Shields of cotton-wool or aluminium foil, as described above, fit the need most successfully. In the acute stage, however, with granulation tissue and/or purulent discharge, there is no place for conservative treatment. The prime need in this stage is relief of pressure by removal of the whole or part of the nail, and when the infective process has been brought under control and a new nail growing, the soft tissues can be protected from its advancing margin by the above conservative methods.

OS CALCIS SPUR

SYMPTOMS

The patient, who is usually overweight and in the second half of life, complains of pain under the heel, worse on standing. In some of these patients, the maximal tenderness is under the heel at the position of the medial tubercle of the os calcis. These patients could possibly be considered as having an os calcis spur, but one must beware of assuming that the spur is the cause of the patient's symptoms. It is common, on X-ray, to find an os calcis spur when the patient is free from symptoms and it is equally common to find a patient with symptoms at this site in whom no spur is visible on X-ray. Indeed, the writer has seen one case of a patient who complained of pain at the correct site with no spur visible on X-ray, but a spur was present on the contralateral painless foot.

TREATMENT

When the practitioner is convinced that the symptoms are due to the presence of an os calcis spur, it is reasonable to relieve this area of the trauma of weight-bearing. This can only be done by providing an alternative surface for the patient to stand on. Three simple measures are available:

(1) *A ring pad.* This consists of an oval pad of sponge rubber, cut away at the tender site and fixed inside the heel of the shoe. The pad must be of such a thickness that when the patient is taking full weight on the heel, it does not compress sufficiently to allow the skin at the tender area to rest on the inner aspect of the shoe. This appliance works very well for a short period.

The two main difficulties which arise are: (*a*) The pad itself deteriorates with wear unless it is covered with leather. (*b*) The surfaces of the heel become oedematous at the point at which they are not supported and this, in itself, may cause discomfort. The oedema may even increase in size sufficiently to transmit weight.

(2) *A horseshoe heel-pad.* This consists of sponge rubber, preferably mounted on an insole and covered with leather. It extends round the margins of the heel so that weight is not taken on the painful area. It is, in function, very similar to the ring pad, but because one side is open the problems of oedema do not arise.

(3) *Rose's insole.* Using this appliance (*see* Fig. 84, p. 108), weight is relieved over the complete plantar surface of the heel and is instead transmitted through the tissues under the arch of the foot. This is more comfortable to wear than either of the above-mentioned appliances, but is less easy to provide in the consulting-room.

OS CALCIS EXOSTOSIS

SYMPTOMS

The patient complains of a painful swelling of the heel which produces rubbing on the top line of the shoe. This is more common in females, but when occurring in males, is more troublesome because of the firmer stiffening in the shoes.

PATHOLOGY

Clinical examination and X-ray will usually reveal that the posterior margin of the os calcis immediately above the insertion of the tendo-Achilles, is more prominent than usual. This prominence produces rubbing between the skin and the heel of the shoe, resulting in oedema and work hypertrophy of the skin which, therefore, increases the pressure and makes the rubbing worse.

TREATMENT

(a) *Raising the heels of the shoes* encourages the foot to slide forward in the shoe, thus avoiding rubbing against the heel. This is a simple solution and females will often say spontaneously that they are more comfortable in high heels. One difficulty, however, is that the heel of the shoe is carefully shaped to follow the contours of the wearer's heel and if the heel height is increased by perhaps ½ inch (1·25 cm.) in that shoe, the top line will cut into the foot in the region of the tendo-Achilles. It is wiser to suggest that the patient should buy a new pair of shoes with a heel higher than that already worn.

(b) *Rubber heel-grips.* If thin strips of rubber are bought and fixed with adhesive to the inner aspect of the shoe, having been carefully cut away to avoid the traumatized area, this will frequently move the foot forward in the shoe sufficiently to avoid the tender region (*see* Fig. 99, p. 138).

In summary, then, either of the above methods can be expected to produce some improvement in a minor state, but in the well-defined condition, they are more useful as post-operative appliances to prevent a recurrence.

WINTER HEEL
(Sub-Achilles bursitis)

This is a condition of inflammation occurring in the sub-Achilles bursa, usually in females, and more common in the winter. It responds readily to the measures outlined for os calcis exostosis.

SUPERFICIAL ACHILLES BURSITIS

Patients, who are usually young females, are occasionally seen with swelling of the superficial tissues immediately proximal to the insertion of the Achilles tendon. These patients have inflammation and effusion into a superficial bursa overlying the Achilles tendon. This responds readily to the measures outlined for os calcis exostosis.

SIX

Adaptations of Footwear

THE NORMAL SHOE

Shoes were probably first used as protection against stones, thorns and small animals. Since then they have passed through several stages, being at times mainly decorative, then status symbols, and most recently, a sort of uniform to show the social group into which many teenagers place themselves.

Excluding special types of footwear, such as climbing boots and ballet shoes, a number of common features can be found. The sole of the shoe is obviously protective in function and its outline is meant to conform to the shape of the foot when weight-bearing but allowing some latitude for style. The upper holds the foot in contact with the sole of the shoe, more or less securely. The height and shape of the heel varies considerably with fashion, this being more noticeable in ladies' shoes.

BASIC PLAN OF THE SHOE

Wood-Jones goes into considerable detail in his excellent book entitled *Principles of Anatomy as seen in the Human Foot* to describe the relative lengths of metatarsals and phalanges, stating that in the majority of people, the first digital ray is longer than the others. Several writers have questioned his views saying that a relatively large proportion of normal feet have the second ray at least as long as the first. Examination of shoes suggests that the latter statement is accepted most readily by the majority of manufacturers.

Many writers have discussed the position of the big toe relative to the line of the first metatarsal and most of these accept that a valgus displacement of up to 10 degrees is within normal limits in the adult and manufacturers have again made use of this deviation to produce a shoe which is aesthetically more pleasing.

In assessing the fit of a shoe, one must first take into account the length and width of the foot. This can be not only measured directly but compared with a shoe by placing the subject's heel into the heel of the shoe and the forefoot lying on the surface of the upper. On insertion of the foot into the shoe, one must feel for areas of localized pressure, both when weight-bearing and non-weight-bearing. The grip of the patient's heel by the footwear must be assessed and also the method of holding the shoe on to the foot (see below). Adequate room must be available in the toe of the shoe to allow movement and there should be no undue tension across the front of the shoe.

The anterior transverse arch is known to flatten during weight-bearing and when walking on a level surface in bare feet the metatarsal heads lie on the same horizontal plane. It is not uncommon to find shoes in which the pedal surface of the sole is concave, and during weight-bearing there must be a complete reversal of the anterior arch, resulting in stretching of the anterior intermetatarsal ligaments, broadening of the foot, pes planus anterior and clawing of the toes, with development of corns and bunions.

CONSTRUCTION OF THE UPPERS

The part of the upper which lies over the metatarsals and toes is termed the vamp. It is the usual site for lacing or other form of fixation. Tension applied at this site (e.g. by tying laces) pulls the waist of the shoe round the shafts of the metatarsals, increasing the constriction which is already present behind the metatarsal heads, thus fixing the foot within the shoe. The constriction mentioned above is even more important when lacing is not used (e.g. in court shoes) and it is in this type of footwear that the waist of the shoe is most marked.

QUARTERS AND COUNTERS

The quarters are that part of the upper which surrounds the wearer's heel and this is frequently reinforced by stiffening termed 'counters'. With shoes which have some form of fixation, the counters can be fairly loose but in court shoes it is essential that they fit firmly against the subject's heel and grip it to prevent the heel riding out of the shoe with each pace forward.

HEEL HEIGHTS

The use of a high heel probably began for aesthetic reasons as the shortened calf muscle produces a more graceful curve of the leg. The disadvantage is that prolonged wear of high heels produces adaptive contracture of the calf muscles and posterior tissues of the ankle joint, thus causing aching when the subject reverts to lower heels.

In an attempt to produce a graceful shoe outline, most high heels today are shaped so that the anterior margin flows into the arch of the shoe. In previous fashions the 'knock on' heel was used, in which the upper and sole were assembled and the heel simply added afterwards.

In all high-heeled shoes it is necessary to add a stiffener to support the arch of the shoe and this stiffener may consist of either a strip of wood which is usually straight in its length or, in the more expensive shoes a curved strip of metal. In the former case, the sole of the shoe is extended backwards in a straight line from the metatarsal heads, rising to a height which varies with the height of the intended heel. Thus, when worn, the inner aspect of the shoe forms a slope down which the wearer's foot slides, thus leading to cramping of the toes in the shoe and this cramping is only limited by pressure of the foot against the top line of the shoe (*see* Fig. 93).

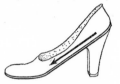

Fig. 93. High-heeled shoe with straight stiffener

In those shoes which have a metal stiffener, it is possible for this to be curved so that the metatarsal heads and the os calcis both rest on a horizontal surface but one raised above the other by the height of the heel; this means that there is no tendency towards cramping of the toes but, unfortunately, owing to extra manufacturing manipulations necessary, this type of shoe is inevitably more expensive than those which carry a wooden stiffener (*see* Fig. 94).

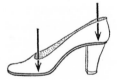

Fig. 94. High-heeled shoe with curved stiffener

The ability to wear a high heel depends partly on free dorsiflexion of the first metatarsophalangeal joint. Even when standing, the angle of dorsiflexion at the first metatarsophalangeal joint equals the pitch of the shoe but at each pace forward further dorsiflexion is produced passively as the shoe bends across the vamp. It is obvious, therefore, that any degenerative change which limits movement of this joint will limit the choice of heel heights.

Fusion of the first metatarsophalangeal joint is sometimes carried out for a number of conditions and the angle of fusion must be carefully chosen, bearing in mind the height of the heels customarily worn.

DEFORMITIES AND FOOTWEAR

It is almost impossible to find in the literature a description of the normal foot. Many attempts have been made but there are so many factors to be considered that satisfactory criteria have not yet been enumerated. For example, the upper limit of valgus deviation of the big toe has been put as high as 25 degrees but the majority of writers consider that 10 degrees is the upper limit of normal. Also, the angle formed between the axis of the first and second metatarsals has been the subject of great controversy and again, most writers accept 10 degrees as the maximum normal.

There is no doubt that a great many commercially available shoes tend to push the toes into an angle of valgus which exceeds 10 degrees and with the advent of pointed shoes, which were used a few years ago, this tendency was produced to its most extreme.

Apart from perpetuating, or even producing, the above mentioned deformities, the development of corns over bony prominences is extremely common. It is accepted by most authorities that a corn is the result of pressure and friction occurring over bony prominences with a small gap between them. Tight shoes, therefore, produce just this set of circumstances and it is common to see patients with eight corns on each foot over the interphalangeal joints of the lateral four toes. Simple instruction regarding footwear will allow these abnormalities to subside without further treatment and there is little point in excising corns unless the patient is prepared to purchase correctly fitting shoes.

Almost as important as shoe size in preventing deformities of the feet is stocking size and it is common to find patients whose shoes fit but whose stockings are at least one size too small.

THE NORMAL SHOE

Reduced to its simplest form, the correct shoe is one that fits, and fit is determined by:

(*a*) Adequate room for the toes while weight-bearing.

(*b*) Adequate width at the broadest part of the foot while weight-bearing

(*c*) A method of holding the shoe to the foot in such a way that the two function as a single unit. This is relatively easy to achieve with lace-up shoes since the space necessary to put the foot in can be reduced after application. Court shoes, however, are more difficult in that the only possible method of retaining the shoe is a firm grip around the counters and pressure behind the first metatarsal heads provided by the constriction at the waist of the shoe. It is obvious that the smaller the area of heel in contact with the ground, the more firmly must the shoe grip the foot. It follows, therefore, that the fit of the shoe with a stiletto heel must be more accurate than with brogues. Straps across the metatarsal bases form an excellent method of retaining the shoe on the foot, although there is not the infinite variation of size which can be achieved with lacing. Straps passing round the heels, as seen in the 'sling back' shoes popular some years ago, rely on tightness and forcing the foot into the toe of the shoe to achieve retention, but, because of the lack of control between the heel of the shoe and the strap passing round the Achilles tendon, it is often difficult to keep the heel under the centre of gravity when walking.

EXAMINATION OF THE SHOE

No examination of a patient complaining of painful or deformed feet is complete without inspection of the footwear. A pair of shoes not recently mended must be available and there are many points to be considered.

INSPECTION OF UPPERS

An alteration of line of weight-bearing in the foot is frequently indicated by deviation of the top line of the shoe. Inspection of a new pair of shoes shows that the top line forms an oval through which the foot is inserted and the greatest dimension of this oval is parallel to the mid-line of the shoe.

In planovalgus deformities, it is common for this oval to be displaced towards the medial side anteriorly and, in an extreme case, this deviation might amount to 25 degrees. Accompanying this, one can often see horizontal creases on the medial border of the shoe at about the level of the necks of the metatarsals and this is further evidence that the antero-medial part of the shoe has been subjected to abnormal weight-bearing. The posterior seam will often give a similar indication, being deflected towards the medial side at the top line (*see* Fig. 95).

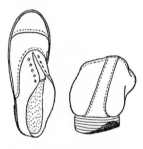

Fig. 95. Deformation of shoe in planovalgus foot

The deposition of the transverse creases across the vamp of the shoe gives some indication of the amount of dorsiflexion which occurs at the metatarsophalangeal joints when walking.

INSPECTION OF THE SOLES

If the pair of shoes are placed on a level surface and examined together, one can often estimate the degree of eversion of the feet in a planovalgus deformity on inspection of the sole. Many of the shoes seen in hospital practice today have composition soles, or perhaps adhesive rubber soles, and these all bear a pattern on their surface. Inspection of the remnants of this pattern give a clue to the lines of weight-bearing when walking and will often provide a guide to corrective measures necessary. This wear can be less readily estimated in leather-soled shoes since there is no true surface pattern but the author has experimented with rubber soles made of alternate layers of black and white, which give not only a pattern of weight-bearing, but can be used to estimate the degree of weight-bearing at any particular point since the thickness of the respective layers is known. It has been found by this method and comparison with footprints taken, as described by Harris and Beath, that shoe wear does accurately mirror the weight-bearing pattern of the bare feet when walking. This is obviously to be expected and unless one takes footprints of every patient complaining of difficulties of walking, examination of the shoe is the only adequate means of assessing the walking pattern (*see* Fig. 96).

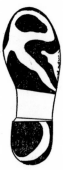

Fig. 96. Wear of a laminated sole

THE USE OF INSOLES IN FOOTWEAR

The great majority of insoles prescribed are of the passive supporting nature. In other words, they act as a 'prop' to a particular part of the foot. This prop may be used for relief of excessive weight-bearing in localized parts of the foot or may be used to correct the position of application of the foot to the ground, but the mechanism of function is the same in either case.

Insoles can be applied effectively to shoes which have a heel height of less than $1\frac{1}{2}$ inches (3·75 cm.). If used in shoes exceeding this level, the slope of the tarsal and metatarsal area of the shoe is so great that sliding between the foot and the insole or the insole and the shoe is inevitable. Also, it is not possible with this position of the foot to relieve weight from the first metatarsal heads by pressure under their necks. Therefore, if insoles are to be provided, the first essential is to check that the heel height does not exceed a practical level.

Since the insoles are of the passive supporting variety, they will tend to maintain, or even increase either the longitudinal or anterior transverse arch of the foot, or perhaps both. If the patient is suffering from pes planus anterior, the arch will have flattened and the forefoot broadened. By reforming the arch, the distance between the first and fifth metatarsal heads in the straight line will be reduced and, therefore, the foot becomes narrower. The same argument holds good for an appliance which maintains the longitudinal arch, resulting in a shorter foot. Therefore, as far as shoe length and width are concerned, there is no need for an increase in shoe size when insoles are worn.

However, restoration of either of the arches does tend to increase foot height and it may well be that with a given foot and a rigid opening, discomfort will be produced by this increase. If the patient has shoes with elastic inserts or of a lace-up variety, this increase in height can readily be accommodated but with the more rigid type of shoe, some difficulty may be produced. This may also be seen when an elevated insole is used in the heel of a shoe to correct a deficiency in leg-length.

There is a tendency during walking for insoles to move about within the shoe, particularly if the method of fixation of the shoe to the foot is not fully efficient. Even with full length insoles there is a tendency for them to move posteriorly and one frequently finds that the extreme posterior margin of the insole rides up the heel of the shoe, thus the functional part of the appliance is displaced posteriorly and its efficiency may be impaired. To prevent this movement of the appliance, it is important that the shape of the appliance should conform to the shape of the inner surface of the shoe and thus it is necessary for a patient to have insoles for each pair of shoes. If this is to be provided, the possibility of movement can be considerably reduced by sticking the insole in position.

CARE OF INSOLES

If not fixed to the shoes, insoles should be removed at night. They should be dressed with leather softeners to keep them supple, and before insertion into the shoe, both surfaces should be lightly dusted with talcum powder.

ADAPTATIONS TO FOOTWEAR

MEDIAL OR LATERAL WEDGES

These may be applied to the heel, sole, or both together. They are best inserted below the surface layer of the sole of the shoe to facilitate repair of the shoe at a later stage. The customary height of the maximum is between an eighth and a quarter of an inch.

An extreme variety of this is seen in the spider boots which used to be prescribed for talipes equino-varus. These consisted of an oval sole-plate screwed to the sole and heel of the shoe. Projecting from the lateral margin of this were two vertical bars which exceeded the two on the medial side by $\frac{1}{4}$ inch (0·6 cm.) to $\frac{1}{2}$ inch (1·25 cm.). Their extremity was welded on to the surface of an oval metal plate, curved in its antero-posterior plane to provide a rocker effect. Thus, the subtaloid joint was subjected to a marked eversion strain at each pace taken by the child and thus, the tight medial structures of the foot were stretched at each step. The children became remarkably adept at coping with these appliances, which must, of course, be used bilaterally because of the increased height although eversion should only be given on the affected side. The appliance, however, does put considerable strain on the structure of the shoe and there is a great deal of damage to carpets and other forms of floor covering in the house.

FLOATED HEELS

This alteration to the heel of the shoe consists of extending the heel in an appropriate direction. Thus, in a patient with frequent inversion strains of the foot, the heel of the shoe can be prolonged laterally, thus increasing the support on that side and tending to throw the foot into a plantigrade position.

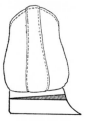

Fig. 97. Floated and wedged heel

Similarly, in a child with marked in-toeing, prolongation of the heel in a postero-medial direction will tend to rotate the foot externally on heel strike. A combination of medial wedging and postero-medial floating is often helpful in the later stages of an in-toeing deformity.

ELONGATED HEELS (Thomas heel)

This consists of an extension of the heel of the shoe under the medial arch of the foot. It is helpful in a patient with marked planovalgus deformity who deforms his shoe so that the instep

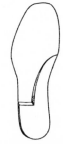

Fig. 98. Thomas heel

approaches the floor. The extra support provided prevents the shoe breaking at this level and, together with the use of a valgus insole, will often maintain an arch more effectively than the insole alone (*see* Fig. 98).

METATARSAL BARS

This appliance consists of one or two layers of leather applied to the surface of the sole of the shoe in a curved fashion to lie immediately behind the heads of the metatarsals. The appliance is usually prescribed for pes planus anterior or metatarsalgia. It is difficult to see how this appliance can function unless it deforms the sole of the shoe. When this occurs, it undoubtedly raises a ridge on the inner aspect of the shoe and this, in turn, may elevate the metatarsal heads by providing further support under the metatarsal necks. The difficulty, however, is that accurate placing of the bar is impossible and certainly much less likely to succeed than the provision of a metatarsal insole. Secondly, the bar readily wears away to lie at the same level as the sole of the shoe immediately in front of it and the elevating effect is therefore lost. It does seem unnecessarily difficult to treat pes planus anterior by provision of a raise to the outer aspect of the shoe when the metatarsal insole can be applied so readily (*see* Fig. 85, p. 109).

ROCKER SOLES

This appliance consists of extra layers of leather being applied to the whole of the sole of the shoe in such a way that the greatest thickness is present under the metatarsal heads, the sole tapering away to either side. The sole at its thickest point is usually at least $\frac{1}{2}$ inch (1·25 cm.) thick, but the extra strengthening provided and the increased curve of the outer surface of the sole ensures that bending of the shoe across its mid-point is not only prevented, but becomes unnecessary. The sole of the shoe then takes on the same shape as that seen in clogs. It is used particularly in a patient who has a painful hallux rigidus,

and avoids the need for dorsiflexion at the first metatarsophalangeal joint at each pace forward. The increased thickness
of the sole is such, however, that it is advisable to raise the heel
of the shoe by a similar amount to avoid the need for the
patient to stand in calcaneous. This adds a considerable amount
to the weight of the shoe and it is quite an unsuitable appliance
to be provided for women except for those who wear the
heaviest type of brogues (*see* Fig. 74, p. 94).

STEEL SOLE PLATE

Insertion of a strip of steel running from the heel of the shoe
to the tip between the layers of the sole has been described to
avoid the need for dorsiflexion of the first metatarsophalangeal
joint. There is no doubt that the provision of this appliance
will indeed avoid the unwanted movement, but the axis of
hingeing of the foot is displaced forwards from the level of the
metatarsal head to the tip of the shoe. This greatly increases
the effort of walking heel-to-toe and a patient with this
appliance is usually seen to walk with his hips externally
rotated, rolling from his heel to the medial border of the shoe,
thus avoiding the more difficult heel-toe gait. There is subsequent loss of grace and agility. If one desires to maintain
the normal gait and still prevent dorsiflexion of the first
metatarsophalangeal joint during walking, a rocker sole would
be much more suitable.

HEEL RAISE

Inequalities of the lower limb up to $\frac{3}{4}$ inch (3·75 cm.) can be
compensated quite satisfactorily by alteration to the height of
the heel of the shoe. This may be done solely by the addition of
layers of leather to one heel or by partial reduction on the other
side. When raising the heel of the shoe, one must remember
that the sole must still be in contact with the ground when
standing, and, therefore, the posterior border of the heel has to
be raised more than the anterior border. The effective height

of the raise is that height which is present under the posterior border of the patient's heel, i.e. approximately $\frac{3}{8}$ inch (0·95 cm.) in front of the posterior margin of the heel of the shoe. The requested height must be adjusted to take this into account. The fitter making the alteration should be requested to add the extra layers at some point away from the under-surface of the heel and these deep layers should be chamfered to produce the increase in height required while keeping the sole of the shoe on the ground. Placing the chamfered layers some distance from the heel surface ensures that subsequent repairs can be carried out without difficulty.

A small wedge insole in the shoe can often be provided to give an extra $\frac{1}{4}$ inch (0·6 cm.) or $\frac{3}{8}$ inch (0·95 cm.) raise. This is quite satisfactory in lace-up shoes, but when the patient habitually wears court shoes, there is a great tendency for the heel to lift out of the shoe at each pace forward. This may be prevented by using heel-grips, which are thin strips of rubber with corrugations on the surface, stuck to the inner aspect of the counters of the shoe.

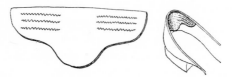

Fig. 99. Rubber heel grip

A Summary of Conditions Requiring Appliances

(For individual appliances see List of Figures on pp. 6 and 7)

UPPER LIMB LESIONS

LOWER LIMB LESIONS

FOOT APPLIANCES